IN SUPPORT OF FAMILIES

In Support of Families

*

Edited by

MICHAEL W. YOGMAN and

T. BERRY BRAZELTON

Harvard University Press
Cambridge, Massachusetts
London, England

This book is printed on acid-free paper, and
its binding materials have been chosen
for strength and durability.

Library of Congress Cataloging-in-Publication Data
In support of families.

    Bibliography: p.
    Includes index.
    1. Family—United States—Congresses. 2. Family—
United States—Psychological aspects—Congresses.
3. Stress (Psychology). I. Yogman, Michael W.
II. Brazelton, T. Berry.
HQ536.I5 1986   306.8′5   86-9855
ISBN 0-674-44735-2 (alk. paper)

*

Contents

IN SUPPORT OF FAMILIES

MICHAEL W. YOGMAN and
T. BERRY BRAZELTON

The Family,
Stressed yet Protected

IF WE VIEW the family as a system interacting with other
social systems, we can better understand the influence of stresses
and supports on child development. A systems approach is becoming popular in the biological and behavioral sciences: it is a concept
borrowed from engineering where precise mathematical manip-
ulation has used systems concepts (such as feedback control) to
develop products (such as thermostats). Philosophers and biolo-
gists—Ludwig von Bertalanffy, Claude Bernard, Walter Cannon—have successfully applied general systems theory and
homeostasis to explain the regulation of physiological systems (Bertalanffy, 1968; Cannon, 1930). But when we shift to behavioral
systems involving individuals, families, groups, or even populations, we find enormous complexity and lack of precision. Although John Bowlby's attachment theory (1969), with its systems
concept of goal-directed and goal-corrected behavior, has been
extremely useful, more is needed: a fuller understanding of the
complicated, irrational love between parents and child requires
consideration of the multiple, often conflicting goals of each individual within the family. For a long time we have been reminded
of the complexity of human beings, the illogic of the family itself,
and its inaccessibility to theoretical explanation and prediction.
Robert Coles, for one (1985), cautions us to listen to individuals

and not to submit our observations about families to the sovereignty of deified but inappropriate theories.

Why have we attempted to apply the concept of systems to children and families? As a result of advances in communication and technology, today's family is bombarded by more information than ever before and is subject to more diverse influences. A systems theory recognizes the broader ecological forces influencing the modern family, offers a method that maximizes sensitive observation of these influences, and will stimulate better research, better theory, and better social policies for families and children. Further, systems theory allows us to analyze family responses to stress as a disruption of homeostasis that has the potential for learning through reorganization and coping.

In this book we have used broad concepts of systems to find commonalities across the stresses facing parents, such as chronic illness, divorce, teenage pregnancy, and the impact of both parents' working. Previously the theoretical framework and even the very definition of terms such as stress (events versus perceptions) and supports have been vague and unsatisfying, although research is now beginning to add some sharper insights. For example, Gerald R. Patterson (1983) has suggested that the relation between stress and outcome may be different for individuals in isolation—where the outcome is usually adverse—than it is for individuals who are part of a social group. In a group situation, a person may respond to stress by developing more cohesive relationships with others; support from others may mitigate the effects of stress and lead to more positive outcomes. The value of a family is that it cushions and protects while the individual is learning ways of coping. And a supportive social system provides the same kind of cushioning for the family as a whole.

We are in a time of transition, when the boundaries between the responsibilities of the family system and extrafamilial systems seem blurred. In urban industrial society, many former family functions, such as schooling, have been handed over to experts. Hence societal support systems need to be included in any attempt to assess the strengths and weaknesses of the family. On the other hand, our society gives parents a double message: they are held accountable for raising children in today's complex world, requiring special skills and expertise, but the society offers them less access to these skills than ever before. What do individual families need in order to provide their children with the supportive backgrounds needed to master the stresses of daily living? The chapters that follow address this question and focus on three concepts in particular:

(1) A family system is created by its members, and it dominates the behavior of individual members, affects the developmental course of the family, and is marked by the patterns of interaction among members.

(2) The impact of stress can be seen as either a positive or an adverse influence on the family's effectiveness in raising children. It may be a combination of both, but the way the family handles stress seems to be highly correlated with its inner and outer support systems.

(3) It is vital to consider the environmental context in which the individual family system is embedded: its relation to other support systems such as friends, extended family, employment, child care, schools, and health.

The diversity of the current family is extraordinary and highlights the importance of understanding the creation of each family by its members and the influence of family structure on coping with stress. Not only is dependence on an extended family now quite rare, but the monogamous, single-breadwinner nuclear family is no longer the modal pattern in our society. Its prominence actually may have been brief. Melvin Konner (1982) suggests that the middle-class nuclear family of the turn of the century (Freud's "average expectable environment") is most unrepresentative of our species throughout human history. Compared with the extended family of many nonindustrial societies (including hunter-gatherers), the isolated nuclear family is a veritable pressure cooker of emotions, is unusually severe in childhood training (oral dependency, toilet training), and has fathers who are relatively distant from their children. In any case, the social support and cushioning once provided by an extended family have not been replaced by community institutions that can accommodate all our new family structures, such as dual-career families, single-parent families by choice, divorced and reconstituted families, gay families, and social-contract families.

The developmental course of a family can be thought of as

consisting of a series of stages. The first involves the creation of a system among individuals and is similar to the establishment of any group of relationships. Individual values, goals, and rituals become coordinated with the values and goals of the family culture, which can then be passed on to future generations. Once the family unit is established, the next series of tasks involves maintaining an appropriate degree of order while fostering the growth of the individual members. Each individual must balance a sense of belonging with a sense of separateness; the family system must simultaneously maintain homeostasis and yet allow transformation. Salvador Minuchin (1974) has suggested that extremes of family enmeshment or disengagement are associated with psychiatric and psychosomatic disorders. While all individuals and families grapple with this task, differences in cultural goals may significantly shift the balance toward a greater sense of belonging or a greater sense of separateness.

The concept of coupled systems that has derived from information theory is a useful analogue (Ashby, 1956). The concept of a mother-father-infant triad in homeostasis captures the mutual influences of three balanced subsystems: mother–father, mother–infant, and father–infant. Any disruption of the system allows for separation, differentiation, and individuation for each member of the triad as family equilibrium is restored. Reorganization carries with it the opportunity either for progress or for regression. As Louis W. Sander (1977) points out, systems coupled too tightly lack the flexibility to adjust to perturbations, and systems coupled too loosely lack cohesiveness under pressure. For example, a tightly coupled system might, in the father's absence, lead to a pathological symbiotic relationship between mother and infant, so that the child cannot achieve the necessary independence. Loosely coupled subsystems allow for temporary independence of some subsystems in relation to the larger system. In such a flexible system, disturbances in a subsystem need not seriously disrupt overall stability. Finally, at the appropriate time, a family system must be able to let go of individual members and allow a more autonomous passing on of traditions within the constraints of its culture.

The impact of any stress on the family system can be thought of as a perturbation that requires the system to respond and reorganize in order to cope. In contrast to the idealized view of family life as free of crisis, all normal families experience stress. The variability of stress occurs both at the level of the concrete event (intensity, chronic versus acute) as well as at the level of individual perception. In other words, some events (death or divorce) seem to be more stressful than others, and events perceived as stressful by one person may not be so perceived by another. Much previous research on coping with stress has focused on psychodynamic defenses and intrapersonal resources. Perhaps, as Patterson's work suggests, supportive interpersonal relations within a family represent another resource to handle stress successfully. The degree of cohesion and communication among individual members is likely to have a significant impact on the way a family buffers its children from trouble. This conceptualization of family stress requires a theory that defines family competence and strength, and not solely pathology.

The identification of psychological and social resources (including grandparents and extended kin) for coping with stress becomes a major task for understanding the family's response. In summarizing the effects of stress on ninety-four adult men followed in a longitudinal study over thirty-five years, George Vaillant (1977) comments: "It is not stress that kills us. It is effective adaptation to stress that permits us to live" (p. 374). When stressed, the family is not merely the passive recipient of external forces. It is active and self-regulating; the family system chooses its external social environment, both interpersonal (friends, neighbors) and organizational (schools, hospitals, clubs). In such an open system, stress becomes an opportunity for a family to change its assumptions and its relations with the surrounding world. If external supports can offer the protection necessary for reorganization and ultimate coping, they become positive supports.

In today's society, however, most support systems do not provide the family with the necessary time and opportunity for testing out different techniques of coping. There are far too few supportive networks available for most families in stressful periods. Employment policies have probably the greatest impact on family life of any external system, since they involve an exchange of money for parents' time. Child-care alternatives, health care, schools, and even the legal system can all influence the family in either a positive or a negative manner.

This volume is divided into five parts, all of which illustrate these concepts. The first section provides a generic overview of stress and its impact on the family system's ability to cope. David Reiss provides a theoretical framework for discussing the family as a system and offers creative empirical methods for studying these constructs. Jerome Kagan and Felton Earls focus more directly on the ways children handle stress.

In the second part, the authors look more closely within the family system and examine the changing role of fathers. One of the major adaptations of this generation to stress is that of pressing fathers into more active roles in the family. Whereas the changing definitions of women's roles in society may influence the role fathers play, changes in men's roles may reflect an independent historical shift, with men seeking increased emotional contact with their children (Yogman, 1982). Employment policies and work schedules have often added to the stress on fathers wishing to spend time with infants. A parental-leave policy available to fathers as well as mothers has been suggested as a needed policy change on a federal level that would provide meaningful family support (Yogman, 1983). The chapter by Ross Parke in this section provides an overview of changes in fathers' roles and focuses on direct interaction between fathers and infants. Richard Atkins discusses families where, at first glance, the father's role does not exist (families headed by mothers). He points out the importance of the way the mother conveys a representation of the father, or maleness, to the children even in a father's absence.

The third section takes up in greater detail extrafamilial influences on the entire family system. By exploring the relationship between work and family life, chapters by Ann Crouter and Maureen Perry-Jenkins, Ellen Galinsky, Abraham Zaleznik, and Gwen Morgan illustrate the connections among the family system, the work environment, and child care. Changes in family structure have not been accompanied by changes in employment policies and availability of high-quality child care. The authors point out the adverse effects on worker productivity and on maladaptive defenses taken from the workplace into the home setting.

In the fourth part, Kathleen Camara, John Leventhal and Barbara Sabbeth, and Lorraine Klerman describe the effects of three specific stresses on families: divorce, chronic illness, and teenage pregnancy. We see here the diversity of intrafamilial responses to stress, the nature of family competence that promotes successful coping, and the linkages between social networks and family and individual development. Patterns of family communication seem to be an important common mediator between each of these specific stresses and the family's adaptation.

The final section examines long-range responses to chronic stress on families. Educational and government policies are a crucial part of the social network of the family system. Bettye Caldwell advocates education for parenting as a means to maximize family coping, while Lisbeth Schorr, Arden Miller, and Amy Fine critically analyze the impact of government policies on either supporting or eroding the family's ability to cope. Both chapters point out the need to sustain what seem to be real improvements in indices of child health and family support, in the face of disturbing indices of slippage as government support of families has decreased.

The book closes by highlighting a policy issue for the next decade. American families now expect that they can raise their children to be healthier and happier, but family stresses of many kinds continue to grow. Has society caught families in the dilemma of rising expectations with the diminished availability of resources for support? Our hope is that an extension of the work presented here will provide some guidance to policymakers in finding a way out of the dilemma.

I *

Theoretical Overview:
Stress and Coping in
the Family System

*

THE OPPORTUNITY to understand a family as part of an extended system, and the individual as part of a family system, gives us a new perspective on methods of coping. The ability of the family to help shape coping mechanisms for the individual becomes a powerful source of strength and of learning. It is difficult to assess the impact of stress on any individual within a family without viewing the family as a system. Each member of the family is affected individually by a stress to other members and musters defenses and strengths to meet it. Also, each member is likely to suffer in individualized ways from the stress and to respond differently. Yet there will be a kind of modeling on others' patterns of coping that will affect each member of a cohesive group. There will be strengths offered one another, as well as a group regression and suffering in face of the stress. This needs to be visualized as a group effort, both in its successes and in its failures. Finally, when and if the stress is mastered and homeostasis is again achieved, there needs to be an assessment of the new level of adaptation.

The systems approach, then, includes all of these elements: (1) individual differences and how they function within the family; (2) the disruption that results from stress to one or to all members; (3) the efforts that must be extended to meet the stress; and (4) the costs of having met the stress along with what has been learned from it. Hence an approach to understanding any individual's stress must include its effect on all members of a family system. This volume will attempt to delineate the components of such an approach.

The first part, with chapters by David Reiss, Jerome Kagan, and Felton Earls, presents an overview of stress and its impact on the family's ability to cope. Reiss provides a theoretical framework and a method for discussing the family as a system, describing the way certain families deal with the chronic illness of one of their members. The chapter demonstrates a very different assessment of adaptations when the family system is examined rather than a single individual. Reiss's work emphasizes the importance of seeing the entire family together and of directly observing patterns of interaction. Kagan and Earls focus more directly on stress within families. Kagan examines social class as a marker of stress for parents in childrearing and discusses ways in which culturally specific learned ways of handling stress may influence the family system, particularly when extremes of the child's temperament are taken into account. Earls looks at the relation between stressors and supports in an attempt to understand the genesis of children's behavioral disorders. He examines the impact of a broad range of stresses on children and provides considerable support for Gerald Patterson's hypothesis that stress is mediated by the nature of parents' relationships with each other and with their children.

1 ✳

Family Systems: Understanding the Family through Its Response to Chronic Illness

Dᴜʀɪɴɢ ᴛʜᴇ 1980s, careful clinical research on the family as a system is becoming firmly established. The first findings from this new area of research have been intriguing. However, as might be expected, there is no unanimity concerning the most productive theoretical analyses or the best methods to test the developing theories.

This chapter has four aims: (1) to clarify the reasons for directly assessing the entire family group; (2) to describe several concepts crucial for understanding the family as a system; (3) to describe briefly an approach to assessing families—a quantitative, laboratory-based method for assessing interaction patterns in families; and (4) to illustrate the concepts with data from a study of families of patients with chronic kidney disease.

A Family Group

Working with families, one of whose members has a chronic physical illness, is a remarkable way of perceiving severe stress to families as well as their internal resources for dealing with stress. In order to introduce these issues, I will describe one of the families my team has worked with (Steinglass et al., 1982). The family consisted of a father who was fifty-six; a mother who was fifty; and three children—an eighteen-year-old boy who had well-controlled diabetes, a sixteen-year-old boy, and a thirteen-year-old daughter. One afternoon, on a broad avenue in Washington, D.C., Mr. Saunders (as I'll call him) was carrying out his duties as director of a funeral home. The place was held up by armed robbers and, in a vicious departing gesture, they shot Mr. Saunders through the spinal cord, leading to a complete transection and dense paraplegia.

The family had always been close and well organized around the father as a genial patriarch. The Saunders were seen by all the clinical staff caring for him at the time as a model family because of their capacity to rally around and support this terribly injured man. The insurance companies and rehabilitation training programs viewed the family's ability to cope as exemplary, and both photographed and publicized the situation.

At this point the family came into our research project. We found them quite rigidly organized around a single principle: "let's support father." A home visit about a year after the shooting produced a disquieting and very different view of how the Saunders were functioning. One clue was the rearrangement of the family home. A plan of the upstairs floor is shown in Figure 1: the cross-hatched areas indicate what changes had been made in response to the illness. Downstairs, things were pretty much as they were before. What had formerly been a music room was turned into a room with physical therapy paraphernalia. On the second floor everything had been dramatically changed. Each of the three children used to have a private room, but now the father had been moved with his special bed into the older son's bedroom. An uncle (the mother's brother)—whom we had never heard about despite all the interviewing of this family—had moved in and became very close to his sister; there were even some suggestions of sexual intimacy. We discovered his presence in the family system only by making this home visit. He was occupying another child's bedroom, and the two boys were now sharing the same room. The adolescent daughter was sleeping in the father's old place in mother's bed.

This panorama gave us a sense that the family, organizing around the father's illness, was no longer keeping track of the developmental needs of other members. In fact, the situation appeared

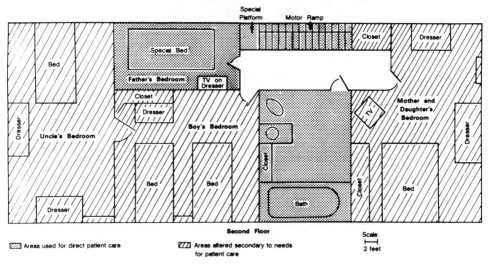

SPINAL CORD INJURY: ADJUSTMENT IN HOME ENVIRONMENT

1. Upstairs floor plan of the Saunders home

quite tragic. This family was not paying attention to the entire system and its requirements and how individuals fit together as a family. Tending to the illness seemed to have life-and-death consequences for everyone. The children had to subordinate many of their own needs—for example, both boys were always called upon to move the father in and out of bed or the car. Eventually their own conditions began to worsen: the older son's diabetes got out of control; the other son repeated several grades and had trouble finishing high school; and the daughter became more and more isolated socially. The family, once highly organized by rules, now viewed the family itself as a tyrant, a disembodied tyrant. Finally, almost inevitably, there was a rebellion. The mother, after two years, decided to take the younger son on the first vacation anyone had taken since the injury. The father counter-rebelled, refused to eat, and, while his wife was away on vacation, developed serious bedsores and was admitted to the hospital. Despite major efforts, he continued to refuse nourishment, and died. The family managed to regroup, and our follow-up showed that the older son did return to reasonably adequate functioning and went into the funeral business.

Data and Concepts

The Saunders case brings out two questions that I particularly want to address. First, when one takes the family system seriously as a unitary group with its own needs, initiatives, and coping skills, what kind of data, both in research and in clinical work, should one look for? Second, what kinds of concepts are most useful for understanding the family as an integrated system of human lives?

For effective observation of the family as a unit, we have come up with four useful guidelines. The first is to *collect data on the entire family unit.* It is unwise to rely solely on the account of one member or even two. Certainly making the home visit to the Saunders family gave us a graphic display of systems principles that we would have missed otherwise.

Second, it is important to *make direct observations.* Researchers should see how the family operates rather than rely on verbal descriptions.

Third, *develop an empathic grasp* of how the whole family functions. In the Saunders family one might see the predicament from the perspective of the paralyzed father, sensitive to all the physical and emotional obstacles he faces; or one might sense the burden and pressures on the children. But it is most important to experience the dilemmas faced by each family member and the stake each has in improvement.

Finally, it is crucial to *note the quality of relationships within the whole unit,* combining direct observation of patterns with an empathic grasp of the unit. Here clinical work with whole families is very valuable.

As for useful concepts in systems work: three assumptions should be made about the family as a unit. First, the family has *initiative.* A family is not a passive victim of outside social forces or unforeseen circumstances (such as chronic illness). The family has its own internal strength and an ability to cope actively. Recognition of family initiative is central to the systems approach.

Second, the family has a *developmental course.* Each family has its own transitional points and its own opportunities for opening up to new initiatives and then closing again. There is recent research suggesting regular, specifiable developmental phases that are true of all families, where they are one-parent or two-parent, whether they have children or not. An early phase is when the family establishes itself as a group differentiated from other groups. A second phase is that of maintaining order while fostering growth of members. Then, often in response to some kind of loss or departure of a family member, there is a phase where the major focus is on letting go and passing on traditions (Steinglass et al., forthcoming; Wynne, 1984). These phases of family development may be just as replicable across families as individual developmental phases are replicable across individuals. And one way to think of the Saunders family is that it was arrested in its development at a point where there would normally be a letting go of the adolescent children and a regrouping of the marital couple. The family, as a unit, was paralyzed: not only Mr. Saunders but the family as a whole was immobilized in its developmental progression.

A third useful concept focuses on *differences* among families. Current research has been effective in delineating differences in organizational style. For example, the Saunders always were a hypercohesive family. Data I present later suggest that such families have a special vulnerability in the face of chronic illness—they get too stuck together. Different kinds of families will handle the same stress differently.

Reference to two studies will add some specificity to these ideas; they will give a feeling of how I and my colleagues used these concepts to guide our observational research experience (Reiss, 1981; Reiss and Klein, forthcoming).

Connectedness among Family Members

My first illustration comes from a series of studies done by our team on multifamily groups (Reiss and Costell, 1977; Reiss et al., 1980; Costell et al., 1981). Data from these observations provide a particularly convincing view of the high level of connectedness and integration among members in a single family system. The use of group sessions is a common intervention strategy in many human-service settings, for a variety of support and therapeutic functions. Ours happened to be on an in-patient psychiatric service, but data suggest that the phenomena are quite general across multiple family groups in other settings.

Multifamily meetings provide an extraordinary opportunity for observing the behavior of single families. Figure 2 displays a seating chart of a family meeting on an adolescent in-patient unit, with adolescents indicated by white squares and parents by black. Typically, these were ninety-minute sessions of from twelve to fourteen families, with one or both parents from each family, the adolescent, and siblings if we could bring them in. To talk in such a public setting is to assert quite a bit of initiative and quite a bit of social power; talking means taking up group time. We asked ourselves a simple question: are families "stable" in the quantity of their talking across nine, ten, eleven, or twelve sessions? (These blocks of sections usually had seven or more families present for the entire time; longer time periods contained too many admissions and dis-

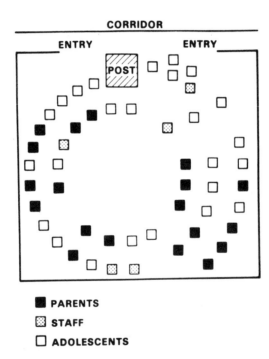

PARENTS

STAFF

ADOLESCENTS

2. Diagram of seating positions in a multiple family group. Twelve separate families are shown, with "adolescents" indicating patients and their siblings. Family members were free to choose their own seats.

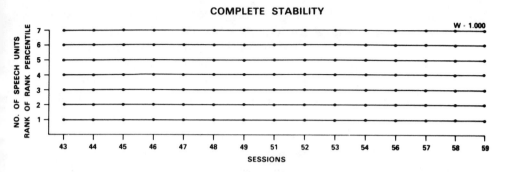

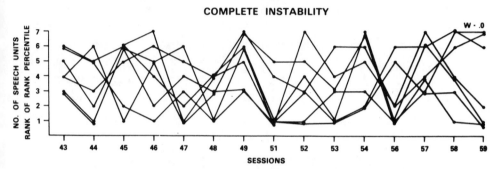

3. Ideal stability and instability participation in multiple family groups

charges to assess stability of participation among families.) Even
as some families come and go, if you track any one family, does
it tend to remain stable, to talk more or less the same over time?
Figure 3 is a schematic diagram to illustrate the data if all families
were perfectly stable—a simplified ideal that will never exist. By
contrast, if families were completely unstable in their use of group
time by talking, they would produce a very random pattern, as
shown at the bottom of Figure 3. We used a coefficient of stability
that approaches 1.0 as families approach perfect stability (top),
and it will be 0 as it approaches randomness (bottom). Figure 4
shows the real data, and we see that the families are actually quite
stable. Those who take up a lot of group time at the beginning
stay at the top; those at the bottom tend to stay at the bottom.
Dividing the data into those from parents and those from adolescents, we see that both parents and adolescents are stable over
time. This stability remains despite a fairly heavy turnover—new

families coming, old families going—across all the group sessions.

Now these findings in themselves are not all that remarkable. They merely suggest that families, like individuals, have personalities; they occupy positions in groups and tend to stick with them. Other data suggest that families occupying either a top or a bottom position have a number of other special characteristics. Families who occupy the top row are internally cohesive and have a clear conception of themselves as an integrated group (Reiss et al., 1980).

Our data from the multiple family groups provide a more remarkable picture of the family as a system. Typically, as Figure 5 shows, what happens in such groups is that parents and adolescents always divide spatially. Sitting apart, they become competitive subgroups. They have their own themes for discussion, and it takes a tremendous effort on the part of the staff to bring the factions together. In this sense, these multifamily groups are intriguing models of certain kinds of community life. The parents and ad-

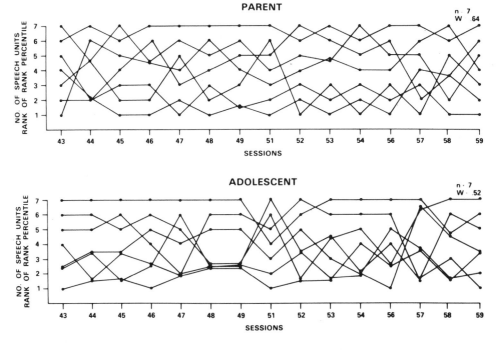

4. Actual findings for parents and adolescents

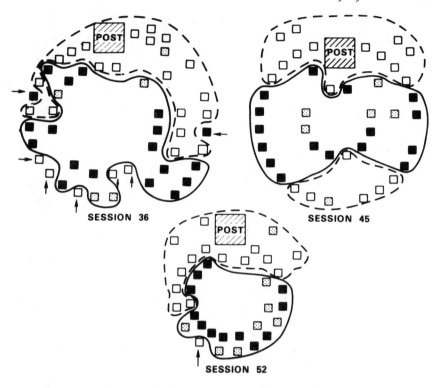

SESSION 36

SESSION 45

SESSION 52

5. Parent and adolescent spatial separation in multiple family groups

olescents seem to be absolutely ignoring one another. However, when the data are examined more carefully, we find that this is not at all the case.

Figure 6 illustrates our quantitative approach to this problem. It shows an example of a talkative family as well as a relatively quiet one and how, in each, parent and adolescent talking rates rise and fall together. This correspondence can be indicated by a coefficient—if the value of the coefficient is high, it means that parents and adolescents in the same family are in close synchrony no matter whether the family is, over time, talkative or quiet.

Figure 7 conveys something quite unusual. Coefficients for many of the families were quite high. This suggests that when the adolescent in this highly divided social system begins to talk a little more in one session, the parents will follow suit. Or it can indicate the reverse: if the parents talk a little more or a little less in one session than in another, the adolescent will soon follow suit. In this instance, what is particularly striking is that this carefully calibrated internal adjustment, shown in many of our families, goes on under a facade of apparent indifference and lack of contact between the generations.

These data illustrate—in very simple form—a basic finding of the system approach to studying families: the intricate and manifold connections among members in the same family. More specifically, these connections are manifested on a moment-by-moment basis. In order for the coefficients of parent-adolescent similarity to be high, parent and adolescent must make changes in a matter of minutes to achieve similar levels of group participation. The

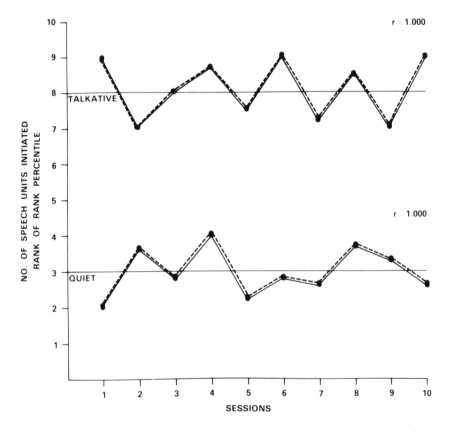

6. Ideal or complete synchrony of parent and adolescent participation

FAMILY NO.	NO. OF SESSIONS	CORRELATION (r)	SIGNIFICANCE LEVEL (TWO-TAIL) ★
6	46	.55	.001
8	34	.42	.01
10	27	.49	.02
11	40	-.051	NOT SIGNIFICANT
12	44	.30	.05
14	44	.30	.05
15	40	.28	0.1
16	37	.42	.01
17	35	STATISTIC NOT COMPUTABLE	
18	23	-.098	NOT SIGNIFICANT

★WITH-IN FAMILY CORRELATIONS DO NOT MEET INDEPENDENT SAMPLING ASSUMPTIONS. HENCE, SIGNIFICANCE LEVEL IS FOR INFORMAL COMPARISON.

7. Actual coefficients assessing parent-adolescent similarity in session-by-session participation

family-system approach rests, very substantially, on this type of directly observed interaction pattern. A new window opens up on family life.

Chronic Illness

How can our concepts and data on family connectedness be applied to understanding families facing a chronic illness? As noted, three basic concepts include the family as initiator, the family as a developing unit, and individual differences among families. The study I cite focuses on the concept of individual differences, picks up some of the themes from the Saunders case, and highlights the enormous differences among families in dealing with a chronic stress (Reiss et al., forthcoming). The group of families we studied was a small one dealing with the same crisis, chronic renal dialysis. Society now is confronted with a tremendous gap between technological advances and a humanistic, interpersonal understanding of what those advances require of families. No condition I know of better represents that disparity than chronic renal disease.

When patients finally come to the point where their kidneys no longer function, modern medicine can keep them alive, not indefinitely but for a long period of time, by a thrice-weekly cleansing of the blood on a hemodialysis machine. There are some alternate forms of treatment that are more family-oriented, but this is still the predominant form of treatment because it is paid for by the federal government. (If that were not the case, the problem would not exist—few families could provide this kind of massive care on their own.) The patient in the family, usually an adult in the mid-years, goes for four hours three times a week to be hooked up to the dialysis machine to duplicate the kidney functions.

Now families in this situation are faced with an extraordinary set of ambiguities and challenges, two in particular. It is not precisely clear to families whether the patient should really be considered alive or dead. The individual is alive by virtue of the machine but otherwise would not be, and there is nothing in the tradition of family life that quite prepares anyone for that. Perhaps more important is the unique nature of the stress on these families. There is a profound disruption of the regular routines that usually keep families connected. There are major dietary requirements, and mealtimes are disrupted in profound ways by hemodialysis. Schedule changes, medical complications, hospitalizations, all occur unpredictably. In dealing with families in this predicament, we have a unique and scientifically precious opportunity to examine individual differences in family behaviors and to understand their consequences, often of life-and-death magnitude.

Most of the twenty-three families in our study had the following constellation: a parent had the illness; there was a spouse and usually an adolescent child in the home; most of the families were black, which is typical of this condition in urban treatment centers; they were, by and large, working-class.

The first diagnosis of renal disease, in our sample, occurred on the average of fourteen months before dialysis began. Data collection started about eight months after dialysis began. We made a second data collection, which I won't describe here, and then did telephone follow-ups at twenty-seven and thirty-six months after the families were first seen. At thirty-six months, almost half of the patients were dead—a somewhat more accelerated course than we had expected; usually about 10 percent of any group of patients on dialysis do not survive after a year. Our research effort was to try to distinguish among these families using three different kinds of measures of family strength. The measures were statistically unrelated, to allow us to account for several differences among families. The research team was fairly confident and hypothesized that high measures of family strength would predict a benign clinical course and long-term survival of the identified patients. Not only were we absolutely wrong, but our data reminded us again that to concentrate exclusively on the survival of the patient, rather than on the survival of the family as well, is a serious error.

The first measure of family strength was done in a laboratory setting we have used for years and involved studying the interaction patterns of the whole family (Oliveri and Reiss, 1981). The first strength we measured, then, is the capacity of a family to stick together when faced with a mild challenge: sorting a deck of cards. Using this technique we could study up to four family members at a time, although most of the families in our study had only three members living at home. Each family member is given a deck; the decks are identical. Families are told to sort the cards into piles, using any system they want. Some recognize that the cards can be grouped according to the patterns of letters on them (for instance, PMSVK can be grouped with PMSMSMSVK). Others use less salient cues. Family members are isolated in booths but can talk with one another on a telephone hookup.

Our interest in this particular task was the extent to which members go off on their own, do not communicate, and sort the cards separately, or whether they make a great effort, as the Saunders most certainly would have, to consult, to check out solutions with one another. This can all be evaluated by simple behavioral measures, very reliable over time. When a family comes back a year later, or two years later, and is given a different kind of task but with the same kinds of measures, their behavior is very similar to that on the first test. This is like a fingerprint or a family signature—the styles are built in. We have labeled this strength *coor-*

dination: the capacity to stick together in problem-solving situations.

For the next two strengths we used more familiar measurements. The second area was labeled *accomplishment*. It constitutes a cluster of variables that are highly correlated and impossible to tease apart: intelligence, measured for each member of the family, level of education for each member of the family, occupational status of the head of household, and total household income. The third area we labeled *intactness*. It reflects the duration of marriage and whether a living grandparent is available to the family.

Our hypothesis was that families would be successful in facing chronic illness if they could stick together in moderately stressful problem situations, if they were intelligent and occupationally successful, and if they had long marriages and support available from grandparents. The actual data had the same kind of reorganizing effect on us as our original visit to the Saunders home: it was the exact opposite of what was predicted. Coordination had a correlation of $r = -.50$ ($p<.05$) with the patient's survival at twenty-seven months and $-.41$ ($p<.10$) with survival at thirty-six months. That is, the more tightly coordinated the family was in its problem-solving task initially, after twenty-seven and thirty-six months, the patient was more likely to be dead. Even after controlling for every possible medical variable, this finding held. It is independent of medical status, severity of illness, length of time on dialysis, duration of illness, and age of patient. The same findings held for most of the accomplishment variables. Intelligence was inversely related to survival, $r = -.51$ ($p<.05$), at twenty-seven months and $-.65$ ($p<.01$) at thirty-six months, as was the level of patient education, $r = -.48$ ($p<.05$), for twenty-seven months and $-.41$ ($p<.10$) for thirty-six months; and household income, $r = -.46$ ($p<.05$), for twenty-seven months and $-.47$ ($p<.05$) for thirty-six months. The more accomplished the family, the more likely the patient was to be dead at thirty-six months. Surprisingly, this is one of the few sets of data in which intelligence turns out to be possibly maladaptive. Intelligence in families is moderately correlated at about .5. That was true here. However, it was the family member's intelligence, not the patient's, that was related to outcome. For example, if the father is ill, it is the mother's and child's intelligence that predicted the father's death, and the higher the mother's and child's intelligence, the more likely the father was to die. The same pattern emerged in the data for intactness. The longer couples were married ($r = -.33$, p = n.s., at twenty-seven months and $-.64$, $p<.01$, at thirty-six months), and the greater availability of a grandparent ($r = -.46$, $p<.05$, for twenty-seven months and $-.64$, $p<.01$, for thirty-six months), the more likely the patient was to die.

What do these data mean? They suggest that we have erred in thinking about death and survival of individuals as the exclusive outcome of concern. The families who find the presence of chronic illness intolerable are exactly those who set a particular course for themselves to maintain cohesiveness, who rise in the outer world in terms of accomplishment, with the intellectual equipment to do so, and who may have intact relationships within and across generations. The situation of illness is a profound derailment of the family's initiative. We now entertain the hypothesis that these deaths were not a medical failure but were, in fact, an arrangement. The patient, recognizing the burden to the family, and the family recognizing how the entire group's interest was being sacrificed, in effect arranged for the death. Now that is a startling hypothesis. But the experience of others seems to support our own informally. We have had researcher after researcher, clinician after clinician, come to us after lectures and presentations, to say "Yes, we see that all the time." In the literature, observations of leukemic children aged three to nine with their families suggest that these children knew exactly what was going to happen to them (Bluebond-Langner, 1978). Three- and four-year-old children knew the difference between an antibiotic and a chemotherapeutic agent, including the names of them. But they would not tell their parents what they knew, because they realized the impact of that knowledge. These children were protecting their parents, and the parents were not attending to this precocious knowledge in their sick children out of a protective wish for the rest of the family. So this death and survival issue has reminded us again that, if one pays attention to the family as a unit, one can have a radically different vision of a process as familiar as living and dying.

Conclusion

I have argued by example, providing some fragments of data to illustrate intuitively the utility of a systems approach. Such a perspective can help to remind us of the high level of connectedness among members of the same family, of the essential requirement to meet the family directly and to look into its patterns of relationships. It should also help to remind us of the substantial differences among families; differences in their styles of interacting within their own boundaries and with the outside world; differences in their objectives and life plans; and differences in how they cope with stress. I have combined clinical material and research data to make another point as well. Our knowledge of family systems, I believe, must be based on two sources. The first is direct, hands-on clinical experience. Nothing substitutes for working with whole families, especially when they are in crisis, to develop an empathic grasp of how the pieces of a family fit together. The second source of data is careful, empirical quantitative research on family systems. This is among the fastest-growing areas in the behavioral and social sciences today, and promises to be a substantial resource to all those who work with families.

2 ✳

A Developmental Perspective
on Psychosocial Stress
in Childhood

AT THE OUTSET it is necessary to make a statement about current knowledge on the connections between psychosocial stress and health in children. It is not stressful circumstances, as such, that do harm to children. Rather, it is the quality of their interpersonal relationships and their transactions with the wider social and material environment that lead to behavioral, emotional, and physical health problems. If stress matters, it is in terms of how it influences the relationships that are important to the child.

Although the general orientation of stress research is to consider unfavorable outcomes, stressful experiences may also facilitate the development of effective, varied coping behaviors, increase personal resources, and lead to a sense of mastery and competence in social development. It is essential to keep both possibilities open to consideration. In this essay I will discuss three related aspects of developmental psychopathology: (1) long-term prospective studies linking childhood and young adulthood; (2) short-term longitudinal studies of children; and (3) the nature of stress and coping in childhood. Longitudinal studies provide a lifespan context in which the significance of psychosocial stress in human development can best be understood.

Long-term Prospective Studies

Although there are a number of retrospective studies in which adults are asked about childhood experiences, my review will be limited to prospective studies because they offer a more powerful source of evidence than retrospective studies. Fortunately, a number of prospective studies have been recently published that provide a much broader base of knowledge than has ever existed before.

Based on analysis of archival data from the Berkeley Guidance Study (Macfarlane, 1938), four generations of families have been studied by Elder, Liker, and Cross (1983). This sample of 214 families, in which the index children were born in 1929, constitutes the most complete source of information about the history of economic and psychological stresses in families. Soon after the study started the Great Depression occurred, and stresses precipitated by unemployment and changes in socioeconomic status could be sharply observed.

The study shows an impressive degree of intergenerational continuity in family structure, with unstable structures tending to remain disorganized across the decades. One of the most important findings of this multigenerational study is the demonstration of how the quality of family relations is affected by historical factors. Negative parent-child interactional patterns that had been established prior to the Depression were amplified as family income precipitously decreased. Fathers were most affected by the economic hardships. Within family units already characterized by poor interrelationships, the transmission of irritable behavior and inconsistent discipline in parents to behavioral problems in children predominated in the area of father and son relationships. The socioeconomic stresses endured by fathers appeared to affect mothers less. The data suggest strong same-sex effects in parent-child transmission of psychological distress. The results do show that predictable relationships exist in terms of the quality of family ties and that hostile and inconsistent patterns of parenting will probably lead to troubled behavior in children (most likely aggressive and antisocial in character). This ultimately gives rise to the same quality of parenting in the children as adults, and the cycle is repeated.

The New York Longitudinal Study (Thomas and Chess, 1984) is a prospective follow-up study from the first year of life to young adulthood. Although the original purpose was to study the relation of temperament to the development of psychopathology, the results point to risk factors other than a child's personality. First, all disorders existing in young adults (average age, twenty-six) could be shown to have derivatives in disturbed child or adolescent behavior. Despite this rather compelling result, it was also apparent that 64 percent of the childhood-onset disorders had disappeared prior to adolescence, and another 18 percent recovered during the adolescent years. Less than 20 percent of the disorders beginning in childhood were still present in the third decade, but there were no disturbed adults who had not been disturbed as children or adolescents. These findings illustrate the significance of prospective studies. A retrospective study, beginning with a sample of mentally ill adults, would have no difficulty in concluding that there is a strong linkage between childhood and adult psychopathology. However, while a retrospective study would imply that it is reasonable to pursue prevention of adult mental illness through the selection of mentally ill children, prospective studies provide a warning that such a process may lead to a great deal of error.

Aside from behavioral characteristics of the children, a number of other predictors were examined. The best single predictor of adult mental status was the presence of parental conflict during the preschool period (Chess et al., 1983). Efforts to improve the prediction by including a range of variables, both behavioral and environmental, were unimpressive. The finding of this longitudinal study reproduces the multigenerational results of the Berkeley Growth Study in which it is the poor quality of interpersonal relations within the family that determines whether a child develops behavioral problems.

A third study, began on the Hawaiian island of Kauai in 1955, examined the contribution of perinatal distress to the development of neurologic and psychiatric problems in children (Werner et al., 1971). The project has successfully followed a birth cohort of over 1000 children to age eighteen. At ages two, ten, and eighteen systematic assessments of the social, behavioral, and academic status of the children were made (Werner and Smith, 1979). By the first assessment it was already becoming apparent that the contribution of perinatal distress was being dwarfed by psychosocial factors. This became increasingly apparent with subsequent evaluations. Boys, in particular, were more vulnerable than girls to chronic environmental stressors, such as marital discord and the absence of a father. These factors also predicted mental disorders at ages ten and eighteen.

All three of the long-term prospective studies reviewed so far have been of normal samples. The next two studies sampled groups that were at appreciable risk for mental health problems.

The first of these is a study by Kellam, Branch, and Agrawal (1975) that sampled black children living in a poor socioeconomic neighborhood in Chicago as they entered the first grade. Here the risk factor for behavioral problems is the stress of poverty and adverse living conditions associated with a deteriorating urban environment. The children were followed over a ten-year period. By middle adolescence, clear sex-specific developmental trajectories were present. The paths leading to dysfunctional status were most easily discerned in boys. Those with aggressive behavioral patterns in first grade had an increased probability of using drugs in adolescence. On the other hand, shy, inhibited behavioral patterns in first-graders seemed to exert a protective effect against adolescent drug use. Anxiety and depressive symptoms in first-grade boys were not predictive of similar symptoms in adolescence, although a weak temporal relationship was found in girls (Kellam et al., 1983). The question raised by this study, as well as others finding sex-specific effects, is how much of this difference is determined by differential socialization practices and how much by innate differences in behavioral predispositions.

The second study employed a sample at high risk for psychopathology because of profound disruptions in parenting during early childhood. This study, carried out by Quinton and Rutter in London (1984), examined the longitudinal histories of female children who had experienced multiple admissions to foster care in early childhood. Despite the stress and adversities of their early years, poor outcomes were not uniformly observed in adulthood. In fact, over half the sample appeared to be doing fairly well in terms of their own mental health and their functioning as parents. These outcomes were attributable to a sequence of successes or failures that began with adjustment to school. Academic and social success in school appeared to serve a "self-righting" function in many of these young women, and this in turn led to a general improvement in their interpersonal relationships. The investigators were able to reconstruct a sequence of experiences that linked improved self-esteem with the eventual selection of supportive men as partners:

Admitted to → Early success → Improved → Ability to → Supportive
foster care   at school   self-esteem   plan   interpersonal
                                                                  relationship

An eightfold difference in the prevalence of psychiatric morbidity was observed within the group: only 4 percent of the women with supportive relationships had such problems, while 32 percent of the women without a supportive relationship had psychiatric problems. Thirty-nine percent of the women with antisocial male partners had psychiatric disorders. This important study documented the developmental sequence that led to the protective effect of having good interpersonal relationships.

From these five studies, certain general conclusions can be drawn. First, although continuity across generations can be impressively demonstrated, there is actually more evidence to support discontinuity. It seems that prediction is most impressively accomplished when the quality of interpersonal relationships in the family environment is considered and aggressive and antisocial outcomes used. Second, rather striking developmental sex differences exist, with males showing greater vulnerability to adverse family experiences than females up to adolescence. During adolescence girls experience a special vulnerability, the determinants of which are poorly understood. Third, variations in marital, social, and psychiatric outcomes within a sample of severely deprived children can be partially explained on the basis of risk and protective factors that develop later in childhood.

Short-term Longitudinal Studies

A number of longitudinal studies spanning a four- to five-year period are available that complement the long-term studies just reviewed. The Isle of Wight Study, the first of these, began by evaluating a community sample of ten- and eleven-year-olds (Rutter et al., 1970). A second phase of the study followed the sample into middle adolescence and found different patterns of change and stability (Rutter et al., 1976). Reproducing the finding of many other studies, aggressive boys had greater stability than any other group. The highest degree of change occurred in girls, who reported a high incidence of emotional problems, primarily depressive symptoms, in early adolescence. This increased rate of symptoms changed the overall pattern of psychiatric problems in the community. Prior to adolescence boys had a higher prevalence than girls, but because of the newly developed symptoms in girls the prevalence rates became similar between the sexes during adolescence. It may be that the earlier vulnerability of males is compromised by a period of increased resilience in adolescence, while the reverse is characteristic of females.

Two longitudinal epidemiologic studies of preschool children have contributed to our knowledge on stress and coping in children, one based in London (Richman, 1982) and the other on Martha's Vineyard in Massachusetts (Earls, 1983). Both studies used comparable methods of identifying three-year-old children with behavioral problems in the general population (Earls, 1980). Once identified, the children were followed over several years. Some 54 to 63 percent of the children with problems at three continued to have problems at follow-up. As expected, boys were more likely to have persisting problems than girls. These studies are of interest because they examine groups of children early in life and then follow them across a significant transition in emotional and social development, and entry to elementary school. While these studies confirm the increased vulnerability of preschool males to psychosocial stress, they also point out how early in life behavioral problems begin and some of the mechanisms involved in how these problems arise (Barron and Earls, 1984).

Supporting the results of these two epidemiological studies is another longitudinal investigation examining the continuity between infant attachment behavior and psychopathology in six-year-olds (Lewis et al., 1984). The findings indicate that insecurely attached males develop more evidence of psychopathology than securely attached males. The quality of bonding in girls did not produce such discrimination.

These studies create a complex developmental picture in which both psychosocial and biological factors seem to influence how children acquire dysfunctional behavioral and emotional states. Both the adolescent and the preschool studies raise questions about possible interactions between the sex of the child and social factors. The high incidence of misery and depression in girls has been ascribed to physical and emotional changes accompanying puberty. In early development, it may be that the slower rate of maturation in boys represents a vulnerability to stress, resulting in a higher incidence of behavioral problems. But cultural differences also play an important role. For example, in the American study (Earls, 1983), the preschool to school-age stability of behavioral problems was similar; in the London study, stability was much higher for males than for females (Richman, 1982). Perhaps this is because of greater parental demands in raising girls in American society than in the more traditional British society. Important cultural differences were also found between white, British-born parents and black, West-Indian-born parents in the London study (Earls, 1982). Although culture-specific childrearing practices were evident, the overall prevalence of problems was remarkably similar in several different populations. This suggests that other factors are involved in the development of dysfunctional behavior. Among the most prominent is temperament. Temperamental characteristics, whether inborn or acquired in prenatal or early postnatal development, provide a substrate for examining more closely how stressful experiences influence emotional development. They represent, in their variety of manifestations, the host vulnerability and host resistance of the child to psychosocial stress and adverse living conditions.

Stress and Coping in Children

The longitudinal studies reviewed above provide a developmental perspective from which the issue of stress and coping in children can be broadly conceived. Although it is important to document the types of stressors that children experience, these studies make it clear that any particular stressful event must be understood within a historical framework. There are at least three aspects to this framework. First, cultural and historical factors create and maintain values and traditions that are manifested in childrearing methods. Abrupt and catastrophic changes in a society undermine these traditions and exacerbate the strains ordinarily experienced by families. Second, these studies find intergenerational continuities in the persistence of unstable family structures. This instability, maintained by parenting failures from generation to generation, is transmitted from parent to child with the suggestion that the behavior of fathers may be at least as important as that of mothers, and for boys perhaps even more important. From this long-range perspective, the contribution of the child to the perpetuation of behavioral problems and social dysfunction in the family appear small. Within a historical framework, intergenerational factors, such as those related to marriage, employment, and socioeconomic status, become the conduit in which a variety of idiosyncratic events and experiences determine how individuals learn to cope with adversity. The shorter-term studies bring the individual child into view and indicate that early acquired behavioral predispositions of the child represent a second factor in determining dysfunctional outcomes. These temperamental characteristics represent either a vulnerability or a relative degree of invulnerability to stress and adversity. The simple accumulation of current stressful events and adverse conditions in a family are not sufficient to predict behavioral problems. The three most important factors are: (1) historical and cultural background, (2) the history of relationships within the family, and (3) temperamental chracteristics of the child. Current environmental and psychosocial circumstances may represent rather minor perturbations in a system understood in this way.

Efforts to improve developmental outcomes take into account these historical, cultural, familial, and individual differences. Yet our capacity to change any one of them is limited. Because both family and individual development are dynamic processes, the most successful tactics will be efforts to redirect undesirable developmental sequences. As health and social service professionals have long recognized, the most obvious points of entry into these processes are represented by a variety of situational stressors and crises in the lives of children and their families.

Types of Stressors

Up to this point a macroscopic picture of development has been surveyed through a series of selected longitudinal studies. What remains is consideration of how more discrete stressful events alter the course of development and, also, present opportunities for constructive intervention.

Acute, transient stressors may be classified in two ways. First there are catastrophic events that lead to significant personal and material losses. Natural and technological disasters, war, and forced migration are examples. The other type of event is more common and consists of changes in health, housing, finances, and family roles. In most research such common events are summated to reflect the total amount of stress and adaptation required of persons over a fixed interval of time.

Numerous methodological problems limit the interpretation of studies examining both types of event. A major difficulty in studies of natural disasters is that it is impossible confidently to interpret negative consequences without knowledge of the person or group before the catastrophe. One of the few studies of children that had the advantage of prior information examined children's reactions to the Boston blizzard of 1978. The consequences of the severe weather conditions were primarily in destruction of property and the loss of valued personal possessions. Findings of the study showed that boys developed anxiety symptoms in reaction to the devastation at a significantly higher rate than girls, and the symptoms persisted for at least six months. Those children considered most vulnerable to the effects of the storm had high rates of both preexisting anxiety and antisocial symptoms. In many, the preestablished symptoms simply worsened: those children who were free of prior dysfunction developed only anxiety symptoms.

Similar results were reported by Milgram (1979), who examined the stress experienced by children during the Yom Kippur war in Israel in 1973. Findings from a pilot study examining the effects of severe flooding in Missouri also indicate the high rate at which children experience anxiety symptoms (Earls et al., submitted for publication). The results of this study show that some of the anxiety symptoms reported are components of the post-traumatic stress syndrome.

Catastrophes are events of great magnitude, involving entire communities or large groups. These massive tragedies can be contrasted with the smaller-scale domestic upheavals that occur in most families from time to time. During the course of an epidemiological study on early emotional development, an effort was made to catalog these events so that their collective and individual impact on children could be assessed (Garrison and Earls, 1983). An important strategy in this research was to realize that the simple enumeration of events with preassigned fixed weights, as is done with the most widely used approach to measuring life events, did not represent a sufficiently sensitive method to study the impact of a wide assortment of events on the emotional and behavioral development of young children. For that reason this project adopted a more probing, biographical or contextual approach in which judgments about the amount of stress experienced in response to a particular event was made after taking account of the biographical context of the family. Preliminary findings indicate that the number and quality of life events seem to matter very little in determining the onset of behavioral problems in young children. Apparently many families cope successfully in responding to transient episodes of misfortune. Adaptive childrearing functions need not be disrupted in these circumstances. On the other hand, families with chronic stressors, such as financial, housing, and health problems, show less evidence of coping, and this measure of stress was significantly correlated with behavioral problems in the children. However, of even greater importance were measures of maternal depression and responses in the children.

There are other studies available that examine the effects of single classes of domestic events, such as divorce, as well as cumulative stress on the psychological and physical health of children. Wallerstein and Kelly (1975) examined the effects of divorce and found in boys more evidence of emotional problems than in girls. In New Zealand, a large birth cohort of children has been followed, reporting a positive relationship between a cumulative index of stress and physical health (Beautrais et al., 1982). The most sensitive measure of stress, however, would not be expected to have any more than a modest effect on children's physical or mental health. It is obvious, whether devastating communitywide tragedies or the more mundane domestic incidents are considered, that most children endure these stressful occasions without psychological or physical harm. This means that the design of research projects in this area has to be enriched, not by finding a better measure of stress but by finding other variables that mediate the effects of stress.

In general, there are two sources of information that provide a context in which the effects of stress can be measured. One source is social and emotional support. Such supports are derived from relationships with significant others and in some cases may be derived from institutional contacts. For children, especially young children, parents and parent surrogates represent the most important sources of support. Parents can either shield the child from the effects of stressful events or help to articulate the meaning of events. But this requires a degree of sensitivity and awareness that not all parents have. Mothers with psychiatric disorders such as major depression are particularly unlikely to be able to fulfill these parenting demands. Thus an important point of intervention is to help parents acquire these skills and to recognize and treat maternal depression. The second type of mediator is present in the child's personality and is represented by a capacity, either learned or innate, to cope with adversity. An adequate research design must incorporate both types of mediating variables as well as a sensitive measure of stressful events. Given the ground already covered in current studies, it would also be desirable to include an intergenerational history of the family in terms of parenting.

New Directions

It may be useful to point out three areas of research that need to be expanded in order to acquire a more complete knowledge on the developmental importance of psychosocial stress. The first regards the need to document the range and impact of stressors from a child's perspective. Second, the mechanisms underlying sex-specific effects of stress must be better understood. Third, the nature of stressful experiences that produce dysfunction must be clearly differentiated from those types of experiences that give rise to competence and good health.

It is all too easy to become convinced that the mature adult view of the world is the right one for all purposes. Nearly all research on the characterization and effects of stressful events in children's lives have been simple extrapolations from techniques and concepts used in adult studies. It is not necessarily true that there is anything wrong with the downward extrapolation of methods established in work with adults to research with children. The problem is to be sure that the child's point of view is satisfactorily represented. It is not sufficient to leave the matter strictly to parents' reports about the quality of the child's relationships, environment, and health status. For example, in one of the few studies of its type, Yamamoto had fourth- to sixth-graders rank a list of life events according to their degree of stress (1978). While many of the events were placed in positions of relative stress similar to those expected by adults, it was revealing to note that certain events, particularly those that registered public embarrassment for the child (such as failing a grade in school), were placed relatively high in ranking. Currently a great deal of attention is being given to comparing parent and child reports on psychiatric symptoms and on conditions within the home environment. Structured, parallel interview protocols have been developed for this purpose. Questions are standardized and as closely worded as possible between the protocols to allow a systematic comparison. Studies using these techniques are in progress; results so far point to wide differences between parent and child for reports of symptoms as well as home circumstances (Reich et al., 1983). There are good reasons to believe that the children's reports are more valid than the parents', especially for subjectively experienced problems (Herjanic, 1984). This is an encouraging result, since better measures of subjective experiences may lead to the demonstration of greater persistence of emotional or internalizing disorders in children.

The second area needing explication pertains to the repeated finding that boys are more vulnerable to the effects of psychosocial stress than girls. There are two limitations to this finding. First, these results are representative of preadolescent samples. As discussed earlier, girls appear to be more vulnerable during and after puberty. Second, what is being termed a vulnerability may be the result of socialization practices or innate differences peculiar to the child. No research study should go too far in one direction or the other. Both windows must be kept open until more is known.

One approach to studying differential sex effects is to examine how boys and girls perceive the same type of stressful event. A study by Emery and O'Leary (1982) provides some insight into this question: they examined possible causal relationship between marital conflict and behavioral problems in children. Children with and without behavioral problems were asked how they perceived marital conflict between their parents. Girls with behavioral problems more often reported feeling rejected by their parents than girls without problems. This was not the case for boys. Whereas feelings of rejection seemed to underlie the evolution of behavioral problems in girls, the process was more subtle in boys. They appeared more likely to imitate their father's behavior during conflictual periods. If the conflict was persistent and the father's behavior consistently aggressive toward the mother, then an aggressive orientation became established in the son's behavior. The researchers interpret their findings to mean that different social mechanisms were at work in determining behavioral deviance. Although different mechanisms are suggested in the genesis of behavioral problems in girls and boys, the significance of interpersonal relationships was apparent for both sexes. No doubt other contextual variables influenced the situation. Yet the study is useful in suggesting how the same type of event produces deviant outcomes through different social mechanisms. It also indicates how simple exposure to an event does not in itself produce an untoward outcome. A parent's active effort to ensure that hostile behavior toward a spouse is not misinterpreted as rejection, or a father's lack of aggressivity in the heat of an argument with his wife, may protect the child from developing a problem.

This brings up the final issue: the differential effects of stressors. Is it possible that the same event in one set of conditions produces adequate coping and psychological strength and, in different circumstances, gives rise to a compromised state of health? There is little scientific basis for answering this question. From the evidence covered in this chapter, the answer is likely to be forthcoming only when acute and chronic stressors are studied together; when we appreciate that current events and circumstances occur in a historical and cultural context that has spanned several generations; and when we recognize that coping and adaptation to stressful conditions are a function both of innate personal characteristics and of responses learned from experience. This constitutes a massive undertaking. Our only hope is that groups of investigators will wish to share these objectives through the use of common methods and collaborative projects.

3 ∗

Stress on and
in the Family

Human beings are continually vulnerable to anxiety, fear, guilt, sadness, apathy, and anger. What changes across historical eras and cultures are the popular interpretations of the causes of these emotions. These interpretations, always influenced by social facts and deep premises about human nature, usually choose one of three origins for the dysphoria—transcendental forces, real conditions, or processes in the body or mind of the suffering person. For example, the high incidence of vagrant youth in sixteenth-century London was blamed on family conditions, especially a lazy father, or on a congenital physical handicap. The same phenomenon in eighteenth-century London was blamed on a lack of parental love and, in the early twentieth century, London psychiatrists assumed that psychological conflict—hostility to a parent or anxiety over rejection—was the primary cause of vagrancy, which now took the form of delinquency and school failure.

In the half century between the First World War and Vietnam a major change occurred in the preferred interpretation of unpleasant feelings. The ideological essence of this change is reminiscent of a recurrent epistemological debate between those, like Aristotle and Aquinas, who believe that the mind is a mirror reflecting what happens in the outside world and those, like Plato and Augustine, who believe that the mind invents abstract prototypic ideas, using whatever slender fragments of experience it requires in order to support the enduring ideal structure. Freud, siding with Plato and Augustine, argued that the biological nature of humans guaranteed that anxiety, guilt, and an Oedipal conflict would occur in all persons growing up in a family. The universal disturbances that the mind imposes on the thin film of real events inevitably lead to personally felt distress and, in those who cannot cope effectively, to a variety of disturbing symptoms. This interpretation of neurotic characteristics satisfied most middle-class adults who, prior to World War Two, did not know that the future would be marred by race riots, civil disobedience by privileged youth, the threat of nuclear disaster, and television scenes vividly depicting the apathy and dirtiness of poverty. But the generation born after the Korean conflict, which was not protected from this information, began to regard their angst as originating not in their unconscious but in real experiences: insufficient love, insufficient money, and insufficient protection from dangers to their health and hardwon property. It seems silly to worry about chronic resentment to your mother when a neighbor's house has been robbed twice in three years and *Time* magazine warns that your drinking water may be poisoned.

When the demons are on the inside, wrapped in mental constructions, we call them conflicts. When they are dancing on the street, we call them stressors. Thus it is fitting that this book has "family stress" as a major theme. In 1950 it would have been "intrafamilial conflict."

When scholars want to explain the normative or universal properties of an entity, they typically look to the inherent structure of the entity under study. We say water flows because of its inherent characteristics; infants become attached to their mothers because of their natural dependence on adults and implementation of species-specific actions that include clinging, smiling, and vocalizing. Only when an entity violates its inherent script—the baby does not attach to its mother—does the scholar look for an efficient cause. Hence, when a person's behavior deviates from what the theorist assumes is normative, the scientist looks for some causal event. In the present historical moment, that cause is often named a stressor.

Stress is invoked to explain maladaptive behavior. Because it is counterintuitive to posit an inherent desire to be unhappy, poor, technically incompetent, or imprisoned, calling upon stress as an explanation presupposes that these reactions are not an inherent characteristic of human beings, but abnormal events requiring a cause. This is a profound supposition about human nature. Most enlightenment philosophers regarded human nature as inherently aggressive, selfish, and cruel and had to explain generosity and kindness. Had John Adams used the word *stressor* he would have applied it to such socialization regimens as a parent admonishing the child for destroying property. Contemporary theorists do not view the young child as selfish, but as affectionate, gentle, and competent. Hence they must explain the child's hostility and failure, but not label the socialization practices of parents as stressors (even though those practices do produce anxiety and anger in children).

Thus the concept of stress has an incompletely disguised evaluative component. Certain events regularly produce anxiety, fear, anger, depression, sadness, and hopelessness. And, depending upon other conditions, adaptive or maladaptive reactions will follow. But we cannot make these predictions knowing only the stressor, say a bitter divorce or an abusive mother. The prediction of future symptoms cannot be made before the fact, only after the fact, for some children react to stress in ways that will facilitate their later functioning. Reconstructive explanations can use the word *stressor* when the end of the story has been revealed, but prediction, which is central to theory, does not have that advantage.

There is, however, an advantage to this outer-directed perspective on development. By focusing on real events rather than on intrapsychic conflicts, we acknowledge that people living in different segments of our society, especially those from distinct class and ethnic groups, experience different stressors. The primary concerns of young ghetto mothers are not the same as the worries of parents living in affluent suburbs. I shall return to this issue in a moment.

Despite class and ethnic differences among parents from different social groups, a majority of Americans from all classes would seem vulnerable in this part of the twentieth century to two chronic frustrations. One is a concern with being loved—loved as a child, as a student, as an adult. A graduate student told a faculty meeting that the main source of unease among his peers was that they did not feel loved. Such a declaration would have been impossible twenty years ago, even though there has been no real change in faculty-student relations over this period. Because love is always a precious commodity, even when it is not in high demand, all members of our society feel relatively deprived. It is not completely clear why love has gained such a position of ascendance. One potential explanation lies with the tainting of the pleasures to be had from status, accomplishment, and power. If gaining the respect of the larger community is sullied—reminiscent of Groucho Marx's statement that he didn't want to join any club that would accept him—then the only other important source of gratification is in a close relationship with another person. Such relationships mute the feelings of anonymity that are endemic in large cities of strangers, and permit one to trust at least one other person.

Further, the emphasis on an intimate relation with another is due, in part, to the increased dignity our society has awarded to women over the last three hundred years. Women in contemporary society symbolize care, affection, and love, and are seen as transcending the meanness of life. Make love, not war, was not just a protest against the indifference and lack of humaneness in Vietnam; it was also a positive statement that love between parent and child, teacher and pupil, fiancé and fiancée, and husband and wife is an activity we should try to pursue in the hours when work is not necessary. It is the one real source of truth, beauty, and salvation in a community where deceit, corruption, and impersonality seem to be rampant. There are very few psychiatrists, pediatricians, or psychologists who do not believe, with John Bowlby, that an unloved child is doomed and that "loss of a loved person is one of the most intensely painful experiences any human being can suffer" (1980, p. 7).

Like most modern commentators on human nature, Bowlby argues that each person has a private judge who sits in approval or disapproval of each day's actions. Whereas Augustine said that God was the judge and Emerson maintained that the arbiter was each person's private conscience, Bowlby puts love objects in the position of evaluator. "In the working model of the self that anyone builds a key feature is his notion of how acceptable or unacceptable he himself is in the eyes of his attachment figures" (1973, p. 203). Although many nineteenth-century observers would have understood and agreed with Bowlby, few would have written three books on the theme because, like the blue of the sky, the idea is too obviously true. Bowlby's conclusions are newsworthy in the last half of the twentieth century because history has led many citizens to question the inevitability of devotion and love between parent and child or between husband and wife. Citizens who question the universality of deep affection and continued loyalty are saddened by that conclusion and are eager to hear a wise commentator on human nature assert that love is an absolute requisite for psychological health.

A second frustration endemic to our society originates in feelings of uncertainty over being unable to reassure the self of its virtue. Each person needs to believe that he or she is a person of moral worth. The Puritan could partially meet this requirement simply by temperance and prudence. In John Adams' time one could simply restrain a selfish impulse in order to feel temporarily virtuous. Inhibiting a desire requires no assistance from other people or from chance. Each person can reassure the self of its goodness and so, to borrow Emerson's phrase, each is self-reliant.

Contemporary American adults find it much more difficult to award praise to the self simply for not giving in to temptations. Indeed, an American twenty-year-old is likely to be teased by friends for excessive self-denial. But, because contemporary adults are not altogether free of the burden of supplying the self with knowledge of its value, they must find a solution. A vocation with status and high economic reward, together with a gratifying love relation, are among the criteria of a virtuous life. Yet one cannot attain these goals simply by willing them. Hence each adult is forced to be more dependent than was the typical Puritan on friends, benevolent authority, and chance for the evidence needed to persuade the self of its goodness.

The emotion generated when someone resists a temptation to violate a standard is characterized by tension and conflict. This is to be contrasted with the feeling state associated with desperately needing a promotion or admission into professional school but being uncertain about attaining that goal. The emotion, better described as anxiety, occurs when the self is not in control of events that can cause discomfort or is unable to guarantee gratification of desires that reassure the self. I do not suggest that the Puritan mood of conflict is better or more mature than the modern mood of anxiety. I only note that historical circumstances can affect the predominant feeling states that are stressful.

To return now to the theme of class differences in stressors. Steven Reznick, Heidi Sigal, and I recently completed an extensive study of sixty Caucasian families and their firstborn three-year-old children. Half the families came from working-class and half from middle-class environments in the Boston metropolitan area. Two women interviewers—Julia Davies and Jennifer Smith—talked with the mothers for five or six hours in their homes. Both child and mother were observed in the home, and we tested and evaluated the children in the laboratory. Let me summarize what we learned.

The mothers of the two classes were different in several important ways. The working-class mothers worried most about aggression and disobedience in the child; the middle-class mothers worried more about autonomy and school achievement. And all the parents were dissatisfied because their child was never as obedient or autonomous as they wanted. This class difference in the ranking of sources of worry is reasonable. Working-class women believe their child must obtain a secure, salaried job and please the employer. An overly autonomous, individualistic spirit might obstruct that goal. On the other hand, working-class mothers also recognize their less-advantaged status and are afraid of exploitation, both of themselves and of their growing child. Thus they experience a conflict between teaching their child to defend the self against exploitation by others while accommodating to the wishes of others. By contrast, the middle-class mother is deeply concerned over her child's academic achievement and future attainment of a professional vocation. Because school achievement requires self-discipline and an attitude of conformity to benevolent authority, the conflict is between overemphasizing a readiness to conform to authority and promoting independence, competitiveness, and individualism. This class difference in origins of tension is revealed in the differential recall of an essay the mothers first heard on tape and then had to remember:

Essay 3: On Restriction

Experts do not agree on the best way to train young children. Some psychologists believe it is important for parents to insist that their young children obey them most of the time. These parents do not allow their children to disobey many of their requests and commands, and they keep a tight control over their children's aggression, lying, and obedience. Other experts claim it is better to allow young children a lot of freedom so that they do not have to do what they are told all the time. The children who are not forced to obey every command live in a more permissive home atmosphere. The arguments for both sides are reasonable. Those who think parents should be restrictive say that if parents do not punish their children every time they disobey a request or command, hit another child, lie, or steal something valuable, the children are likely to become very difficult to control later on and may get into trouble when they are in school. They might become delinquents, take drugs, or get poor grades.

But parents who favor permissiveness say that if children are allowed to do what they want some of the time, they will end up with a stronger conscience. These children will be more responsible when they are older adolescents because they have had practice in deciding what was right and what was wrong on their own and did not behave correctly simply because they were afraid of punishment.

This is a difficult issue to decide. The child who is restricted too much might become afraid to try new things, fearful of his or her parents, and maybe become angry and frustrated. However, the child with too permissive parents might become an adult not willing to do what employers request and not able to work at jobs that are unpleasant. Perhaps the best advice to parents is to decide what actions they feel are important to punish. And for the rest of the child's behavior, parents should try to be more relaxed and, above all, consistent.

The middle-class mothers remembered more of the argument that said a parent has to be restrictive, while the working-class mothers remembered more of the argument that promoted permissiveness. This difference was replicated in several independent samples and seems to be robust.

Many commentators have noted that working-class parents are more anxious and insecure over their personal qualities than middle-class parents are, and do not want their children to grow up with the anxiety created by feelings of intellectual inadequacy and lack of personal achievement. They believe the child must develop the ability to inhibit this form of anxiety in order to gain vocational success and to avoid coercive exploitation. Because they believe that excessive restrictiveness is one source of this anxiety, they elaborate the permissive statements in their recall. Middle-class mothers are also concerned about their child's personal achievement, but their theory of accomplishment maintains that a rebellious attitude and unwillingness to persevere are more important determinants of failure than fear of authority. Hence the middle-class mothers elaborate the more restrictive argument in the essay.

Money is a second important source of uncertainty. Although all young families worry about their finances, the working-class mother's apprehension over feeding and clothing her family is more realistic. This uncertainty can lead to chronic anxiety. As a result, economically disadvantaged parents lose their tempers more easily than middle-class mothers. But display of maternal anger toward a child has come to signify rejection. The family is one of the few settings where anger can be expressed without the inhibiting anticipation of social rejection, loss of status, or counterattack. One spouse often dominates the other, and both parents are always dominant in relation to the child. Society is relatively accepting of the misplaced hostility in a husband's display of anger to a wife which is, in actuality, a reaction to disappointment at work, to difficulties with friends, or to unfulfilled aspirations. But the child, too, is a target for misplaced parental hostility. Because the mother is usually home with the young child more continually than the father, provocation from the child, usually a violation of one of the mother's standards, can release the parent's anger in the form of yelling, physical punishment, or, less commonly, physical abuse. Such behavior is often interpreted as indicating a rejecting attitude, even though psychologists are reluctant to make the same inference in the case of the angry husband. They interpret the husband's anger toward the wife as due to his personal frustrations outside the home and not as a sign of deep resentment toward the spouse. Yet they fail to draw the same conclusion when the mother is angry with her child. Because we find it more difficult to attribute intense anger to women than to men, and believe that the love relation between mother and child is inherently stronger than the bond between husband and wife, the expression of hostility toward a child must require an intensity of dislike far greater than the irritation generated by a frustrating day at work. These stereotypes we hold for the sexes lead most Americans to interpret aggression in men and women differently. Men are dominant or nondominant, women are loving or nonloving. When aggression occurs in men, we attribute it to frustration of their motive for dominance or control of their daily affairs. When the same behavior occurs in a woman, we are more likely to attribute it to a nonloving attitude.

Because economic insecurity is a major source of frustration in the lives of the poor, the uncertainty of economic stress is felt more continually by the working-class mother. As a result, she is more prone to outbursts of anger. These mothers yell, scream, and strike their children more often than middle-class mothers do. This fact is interpreted by some psychologists as reflecting a less loving attitude toward the child rather than as a sign of greater frustration. It is not fair to the poverty mother to add the burden of calling her unloving simply because she is poor.

It is also important to realize that the stressors named by the scholar are sometimes different from those mentioned by the mother. Scholarly essays on family stressors usually mention the death of a love object, job insecurity, family mobility, the availability of drugs to youth, the high rate of divorce, and working mothers. However, when mothers of all classes are asked about what they worry about most, they mention first their own self-actualization and their child's. This discrepancy between the worries that dominate the subjective frame of the parent and those that dominate the objective frame of the scholar does not mean that one of these sources of information is wrong and the other right, but rather that the two are complementary. The facts of possible unemployment and available drugs for youth are translated by the parent into possible dangers for her child's future vocational success. Drugs may sap an adolescent's motivation in school; maternal employment may leach the home of the warmth that most believe is necessary for a child's self-confidence. But the mother's concern with personal abilities, activity, and pleasure is real and not an obvious transduction of the external stressors listed by the scientist. Unfortunately, there is no unambiguous relation between the number of external stressors in the objective frame and the subjectively experienced internal tensions of the parent.

Finally, it is appropriate to consider the effective therapeutic interventions that might help American mothers. The most important actions are beyond our professional power, for they rest with political decisions that can alleviate some of the financial insecurities of the poor.

A second intervention, which is also difficult to implement, involves structural changes in the society that could reduce some of the anxiety parents feel over their child's future. Our society has become extremely zealous in the rank ordering of children from best to worst, much more so than when I was a youngster. Perhaps this is a price we must pay for the morally praiseworthy progress toward affirmative action and egalitarianism and the technical progress that makes it necessary for many more youths to have a technical education. These historical changes have reduced the number of different vocational roles that have dignity and financial security, and have increased the number of young people who aspire to these vocations far beyond the number of available positions.

But professionals can help by communicating some important ideas to parents. Research reveals that 10 to 20 percent of all children are born with temperamental dispositions that lead them to show extreme fear, irritability, activity, or boldness. Mothers accommodate to these dispositions in their children—they do not produce them—and it is not fair for them to bear the guilt that comes from believing they were the sole sculptors of these outcomes. In a recent study Eleanor Maccoby and her colleagues (1984) saw fifty-seven children at twelve and eighteen months of age. The mothers of one-year-old boys who were extremely irritable and difficult to manage had accommodated their behavior to their sons' difficult characteristics by eighteen months, and began to withdraw effort from teaching them because it proved too frustrating. "Mothers of difficult boys were now expending considerably less teaching effort than they employed with easygoing boys . . . The results of this study provide support for the view that characteristics of children commonly labeled as 'temperamental' are influenced by the socialization environment. Although there are endogenous contributions to an infant's initial mood and behavior, they become inextricably blended with the effects of parent-child interaction by the time children enter their second year" (pp. 469, 471).

My own research group has been studying fearful and bold children who were selected at twenty months of age. We followed these children through the sixth year and found that most of them retained their characteristic style. The parents were grateful for the knowledge that these styles were partially temperamental in origin and not the sole result of their practices (Kagan et al., in press).

A second important fact that can help parents is the realization that their child is capable of growth toward health. Extensive review of the literature on this issue has convinced me that the three-year-old child who is showing psychopathology retains a capacity for change, if aspects of the environment become benevolent. In our time, benevolence means a sensitivity to the child's capacities and recognition that the child must feel valued, even if he or she fails to meet the family's standards.

It is important to realize that at each stage of development the child needs different resources from the family. During the first year, variety of experience and the availability of the parents for attachment are primary. During the second and third years, stimulation of language development is critical. During the years prior to school entrance, information that persuades children they are loved becomes critical, and during the school years it is important for children to believe that they can succeed at the tasks they want to master. The half dozen years that precede puberty are preparation for adult life. Young adults must learn an economic skill, accept the responsibility of being a parent and spouse, and assume the duties that come from being a participating member of society. Children in Third World villages help with cooking, child care, washing, and cleaning; those in Western cities and towns learn intellectual and technical skills. During the latency years, American children need experiences that promote academic talents, a sense of responsibility, and, most important, a belief that they can attain the goals valued by self and community. They need reassurance that these goals are attainable. Failure to gain the desired goals produces distress and can provoke antisocial behavior. A farmer in a field teaching his eight-year-old son how to plant corn finds it easy to accomplish this goal. It is more difficult when the child is with a teacher in a class of thirty children. From the child's perspective, the private evaluation of progress is based on a comparison of his or her performance with that of peers. The larger the number of peers used for comparison, the less likely will a particular child conclude that he or she can master a particular talent. A girl with an average IQ and a particular ability profile attending a class of 35 children, in a school of 1,000 pupils, in a city of 100,000 people, will know more children who are more talented than she than will a comparable child in a class of 15, in a school of 300, located in a town of 20,000. This is one reason American children growing up in towns of under 50,000 people are disproportionately represented among eminent adults. The majority of the original group of astronauts spent their childhoods in towns or small cities, not in our largest municipalities with their many resources.

Each person remains continually sensitive to the presence of individuals who are more potent than self, whether the source of the potency is size, intellectual ability, strength, beauty, wealth, status, or endurance. When there is a large number of these more potent individuals, the child may inhibit initiatives that might be implemented if the more competent or powerful persons were absent. Although families cannot easily change their place of residence so that their child can be with children of equal talent, parents can try to arrange the lives of their children so that successes are more likely than failures.

In another historical period, the advice to professionals and to parents might be different. Each of us lives in a historical context and our conflicts are shaped by a matrix of social facts. The reasons for anxiety, anger, joy, and success in Puritan New England are not exactly the same as those that provoke dysphoria in contemporary Americans. Each historical era makes special demands on children and families and promotes special beliefs about the life course. Hence we all impose special interpretations on our experiences. How else can we explain the affection a fifty-year-old Japanese man feels for a father who frightened him throughout his boyhood or the sense of generosity and pleasure a fourth-century Athenian youth felt if he did not enjoy the periods of intimate physical contact with his teacher? The effect of an emotionally significant experience—a father's prolonged absence or a bitter divorce—will depend on how the child interprets these events. Such interpretations are based on the child's knowledge, moral evaluations, and inferences about the causes of his or her current mood. Rarely will there be a fixed consequence of any single event, no matter how traumatic. The puzzle psychologists have been unable to solve is how to diagnose these private interpretations from the actions, statements, and undetected physiological reactions of children.

II *

Forces Within
the Family:
New Roles

*
───

Understanding the family as a system when stressed
requires understanding the changing role of both fathers and
mothers. Ross Parke provides an overview that separates the direct
and indirect influences of the father and examines the impact of
recent historical changes in social context. He pays particular attention to the effect of social networks and supports on the paternal
role. Richard Atkins extends discussion of the father's role in the
family system by contrasting direct involvement to more detached
involvement via letters, phone calls, or merely being the subject of
conversation. First, he discusses the way single-parent mothers
convey the representation of the father to the children in his absence. Second, he criticizes the effort to force direct involvement:
the legal system's attempt to impose joint child custody on divorcing parents too often ignores psychological conflict between the
parents and its possible effects on the child.

Clearly, the father's role in the family system is more likely to
be fragile than the mother's and is more dependent on contextual
influences, both intrafamilial and extrafamilial. Probably the single
most important influence on the father's involvement is the mother's wishes. The mother seems to function much as a "gatekeeper"
in regulating the father's involvement with the infant. The quality
of the marital relationship is another intrafamilial influence on

paternal involvement, and Parke's chapter addresses this. Fathers (as well as mothers) have better relationships with their infants when marriages are free of conflict. The father's changing role is a good example of the internal efforts of present-day families to cope with the stresses imposed by two parents working outside the home. This family readjustment can be seen as a paradigm for coping.

Forces outside the family also have a major impact on paternal involvement. Employment policies and work schedules probably have the most powerful influence of all on a father's role in the family, and the influence is not a supportive one. Policies allowing short-term childbirth leave for fathers or allowing fathers to take days off when their children are sick are very rare (see Galinsky's chapter in Part III). Hospitals have been much more supportive in removing impediments to paternal involvement, and fathers' presence during childbirth has increased dramatically in the last ten years. This shift seems to be associated with positive effects on the mother-father relationship as well as the father-infant relationship. However, fathers are still rarely seen in preschool or school settings. Schools have traditionally been staffed by female teachers, and fathers have in many ways been discouraged from participating in teacher conferences and meetings. More outreach by the school staff is likely to be helpful, but better research in these settings is needed to remove the impediments to increasing involvement of fathers.

4 *

Fathers:
An Intrafamilial Perspective

As the social context of families has changed over the last few decades, the father's role in the family has become more salient and potentially more important for both wives and children. In this essay I will examine some of the ways in which the father's role within the family has shifted.

My first assumption here is that the father's role in the family is most usefully conceptualized within a family-systems framework, in which the complementary roles and behavior of all members of the family unit merit consideration in order to illuminate the behavior of any single family member. Implicit in this view is the concept of mediated or indirect effects of fathers in addition to their direct effects on family members and families. Fathers indirectly affect other family members through the nature of their interactions with their wives and children, as well as directly by face-to-face interactions within the family. Second, there are many directions of influence among family members, with children, mothers, and fathers each influencing other members and in turn being influenced. Third, a life-course perspective is useful because an acknowledgment of the location of adults and children along separate developmental trajectories will assist in understanding the behavior of any family member. The location of a father, for example, in terms of his occupational position and goals will be helpful in predicting his investment in his role as father. Fourth, an ecological viewpoint complements the systems perspective by recognizing the embeddedness of fathers and families within a variety of extrafamilial social systems. (Elaboration of this aspect of fathering is beyond the scope of this essay, but see Parke and Tinsley, 1982, 1984; Tinsley and Parke, 1983.)

Fathers and mothers play somewhat different roles in early infancy. As a number of studies over the last decade have documented (Parke and O'Leary, 1976; Parke and Sawin, 1980; Lamb, 1977; Yogman, 1982), fathers serve proportionally more in a playmate role and less in a caregiving role than mothers do. In spite of their limited involvement in caregiving, evidence suggests that fathers are competent in this sphere. For instance, they are sensitive to infant cues that are important for maintaining the smooth progress of feeding (Parke and Sawin, 1976). Fathers and mothers play distinctive roles in infancy and complement the contributions of each other to the infant's development.

Fathers influence their wives and children in a variety of indirect ways as well (Parke, Power, and Gottman, 1979; Lewis and Fiering, 1981). In this essay I will examine the impact of fathers and mothers as spouses in their role as parents. Although the primary emphasis will be on the father's role as a support figure for the mother, the father as a recipient of support will also be explored.

The Husband-Wife Relationship

Various aspects of the parents' marital relationship have differing effects on the ways in which each parent enacts his or her role. For purposes of this essay, global measures of marital satisfaction are distinguished from specific aspects of support that husbands and wives provide for each other. Four specific forms of spousal support merit consideration: emotional or relational, physical, ideological, and informational (Cochran and Brassard, 1979; Power and Parke, 1984). Relational supports are those that characterize close, emotional relationships and serve diverse functions, from emotional support to recreation. Physical or instrumental support involves the provision of assistance in the execution of the physical aspects of parenting, such as child care or housekeeping. In addition, the provision of financial support would be included in this category. Ideological support refers to the degree to which the spouses support each other's conceptual basis of their roles; for example, agreement concerning the appropriate degree of career commitment for women and men, or the relative child-care responsibilities of fathers and mothers. Finally, informational support concerns the degree to which advice concerning child care and childrearing is available and provided by each parent for his or her partner. After reviewing the relationship between general marital satisfaction and parenting, I will examine briefly each of these specific forms of support and their relationships to parenting.

MARITAL SATISFACTION AND PARENTAL COMPETENCE

A number of studies have documented a positive relationship between the quality of marital satisfaction and parental functioning. (See Belsky, 1981; Lerner and Spanier, 1979; Power and Parke, 1984, for reviews.) Grossman, Eichler, and Winickoff (1980) traced families from pregnancy through the end of the first year and found a positive relationship between marital adjustment and the mother's skill and affection in regard to the infant. Similarly, Feldman, Nash, and Aschenbrenner (1983) found that marital quality was a consistent predictor of fathering involvement. The quality of the marital relationship has implications for infants as well: Goldberg (1982) found a positive relationship between security of attachment and marital adjustment. Similarly, Vincent (1981) found that the security of parent-infant attachment at one year of age could be predicted from observational and self-report measures of the marital relationship at one month after birth. A wide range of studies of older children consistently documents a strong relationship between marital discord and parent-child difficulties (Emory, 1981). In summary, it appears that the overall quality of the husband-wife relationship is positively related to parental competence.

EMOTIONAL SUPPORT

There is clear evidence that emotional support is positively related to maternal competence and role satisfaction. During pregnancy, a number of studies indicate that the husband's emotional support increases and, in turn, is related to adaptation during pregnancy (Colman and Colman, 1971; Leifer, 1977; Rausch et al., 1974; Schereshefsky and Yarrow, 1973). Similarly, there is evidence that the emotional support of the husband during labor and delivery has a variety of positive outcomes for both mother and infant. Women whose husbands participated in both labor and delivery reported less pain, received less medication, and felt more positive about the birth experience than women whose husbands were present only during the first stage of labor (Henneborn and Cogan, 1975).

As Entwisle and Doering (1981) have found, the father's presence during the second stage of labor and delivery increased the mother's emotional experience at birth; mothers reported the birth as a "peak" experience more often if the father was present. The father's emotional reaction to the birth was also heightened by being present at the delivery. In another study, Peterson, Mehl, and Leiderman (1979), based on observations and interviews with fathers, found that a more positive birth experience for the father was associated with his enhanced attachment to the infant. Together, the evidence tentatively suggests that the presence of the father has positive benefits for both mothers and fathers. Finally, in light of the data demonstrating that maternal medication during labor and delivery can have a depressive and disorganizing effect on infants (Conway and Brackbill, 1970; Murray et al., 1981), the father's presence may indirectly benefit the infant as well.

Nor is the impact of emotional support restricted to pregnancy and childbirth. In spite of the fact that the overall level of emotional support that fathers provide their spouses decreases in the postpartum period (Cowan and Cowan, 1985; Power and Parke, 1984), emotional support is related to maternal competence. The impact of the father's emotional support on the mother in her role as caregiver is illustrated in Pedersen's work. He summarized his results as follows:

> The husband-wife relationship was linked to the mother-infant unit. When the father was more supportive of the mother, that is, evaluated her maternal skills more positively, she was more effective in feeding the baby. Then again, maybe competent mothers elicit more positive evaluations from their husbands. The reverse holds for marital discord. High tension

and conflict in the marriage was associated with more inept feeding on the part of the mother.   (1975, p. 6)

Nor is the impact of the father on mother's feeding behavior limited to bottle-feeding contexts. The success of breast feeding has been found to be directly related to the support and encouragement provided by the father (Switzky, Vietze, and Switzky, 1979).

Other evidence suggests that spousal emotional support has a positive impact on parental competence in general and not just in feeding contexts. In a recent study of four- to eight-month-old infants and their parents, Dickie and Matheson (1984) examined the relationship between parental competence and spousal support. Parental competence was based on consistency, responsiveness, and warmth and pleasure in parenting. Emotional support—a measure of affection, respect, and satisfaction in the marital relationship—was positively related to maternal competence. Moreover, in a recent cross-cultural study in Japan, Durrett, Otaki, and Richards (1984) found that mothers' perception of emotional support from the father was related to the quality of the infant-mother attachment relationship. Specifically, mothers of securely attached infants perceived greater emotional support from the father than mothers of anxiously avoidant infants and anxiously attached/resistant infants, "even though the husband/wife relationship in Japan likely differs from spousal relationships in America" (Durrett et al., 1984, p. 174).

Just as paternal support relates positively to maternal competence, there is evidence that maternal support is similarly linked to the father's parenting competence. These same investigators found that maternal emotional support was related to paternal competence. In fact, spousal support was a more important correlate of competence in fathers than in mothers. The level of emotional support successfully discriminated high and low competence in fathers, but failed to do so in the case of mothers. In short, successful paternal parenting may be particularly dependent on a supportive intrafamilial environment. Clearly, support has a differential effect on various family members, and examination of the separate impact on different family agents is worthwhile.

PHYSICAL SUPPORT

Physical support, as in the case of emotional support, varies over time; paternal support increases through the latter part of pregnancy, and physical support from the husband decreases during the postpartum period (Power and Parke, 1984). In contrast, physical support from the social network outside the nuclear family generally increases over time, particularly from grandparents (Tinsley and Parke, 1984). The decline in fathers' level of physical support occurs whether or not the mothers are employed outside the home and regardless of the couple's sex-role views (Cowan and Cowan, 1985; Walker, 1970).

However, women's employment status is an important determinant of fathers' proportionate and absolute levels of involvement in physical-care activities in the home. First, fathers increase the *proportion* of time they devote to the total family workload when mothers work outside the home (Walker and Woods, 1976; Pleck, 1983). Yet this increase often emerges as a result of mothers' reducing the amount of time they devote to housework and child care rather than to an increase in the absolute amount of time men devote to these tasks. These findings are not without significance, since the impact of the father's participation on either his spouse or his children is likely to be different in families where father and mother are more equal in their level of family participation.

Second, there is some evidence for absolute increases in fathers' contribution to family work when mothers are employed, especially in terms of father-child contact (Robinson, 1977). However, this varies with the age of the child, with father-child involvement in family work increasing mainly in the case of infants (Walker and Woods, 1976) and young children (Russell, 1982). Interestingly, the quality of fathers' support is different as well. According to Russell (1982), fathers with employed wives spent more time assuming *sole* responsibility for their children compared to fathers with nonemployed wives.

Finally, the impact of shifts in fathers' participation as a result of maternal employment on either mothers or infants are not yet well understood (Hoffman, 1984). Nor is it known whether fathers' support elicited as a consequence of maternal employment differs in its impact from that support arising from other causes. Other aspects of the work-family relationship merit attention as well, such as the impact of flexible schedules and shiftwork on the father's role in the family. (See Parke and Tinsley, 1984.)

Another set of factors that determines the extent to which fathers provide physical support derives from studies of the impact of the type and timing of the infant's birth. Two examples will illustrate. First, several investigators have found that Caesarean delivery can alter the father's level of participation in routine caregiving activities (Pedersen et al., 1980; Grossman, Winickoff, and Eichler, 1980). In these studies, fathers of the C-section babies were more likely to share early caregiving responsibilities with the mother than were fathers of vaginally delivered infants. Other data suggests that these shifts in roles do not persist beyond the first year (Vietze et al., 1980). The findings, nonetheless, provide support for a systems perspective by illustrating that, when maternal availability is reduced (as a result of a surgical recovery period), the father's level of participation is modified.

A second illustration derives from studies of the impact of the premature birth of an infant on the father's support role. Again, the effect of this stressful event was to increase fathers' participation in routine caregiving activities (Yogman, 1983; Marton, Minde, and Perrotta, 1980). In this case, the increased demands imposed by the care of the premature infant (Goldberg and DeVitto, 1983; Brown and Bakeman, 1980) served to elicit greater involvement by fathers. From a family-systems perspective, this suggests that a change in another family member's status—the infant—can also modify the relative support roles that mothers and fathers play in the family.

Interpretation of these findings, however, can profit from a lifespan perspective (Parke and Tinsley, 1984). Fathers in today's social climate are more likely to be willing to assume greater caregiving responsibility than in earlier eras. In addition, the lessened availability of external support figures, such as extended kin, to provide ongoing assistance in times of crisis or transition may increase the probability of a father's involvement. In earlier times others rather than fathers may have provided the needed physical support. (See Parke and Tinsley, 1984; Tinsley and Parke, 1984, for more detailed analyses of these issues.)

IDEOLOGICAL SUPPORT

For both men and women, adoption of a definition of the parental role which suits their own ideology and the ideology of their spouse is a major task. Evidence suggests that spousal agreement on roles is an important determinant of role satisfaction (Power and Parke, 1984; Hoffman, 1983). Ideological support can have various functions: defining and regulating the relative roles to be played by father and mother, and allowing opportunities to engage in role behavior that is consistent with both parents' respective ideologies.

It is important to recognize that "support" in this context does not necessarily imply or dictate particular levels of involvement. Rather, it suggests that more involvement by the father is not necessarily better or necessarily helpful. In fact, "in many families, increased father participation may cause conflict and disruption as a result of the threat to well established and satisfying role definitions" (Parke and Tinsley, 1981). Evidence of direct relevance to this issue is sparse and inconclusive. For example, Pleck (1983) found that only a minority of women endorse the notion of increased participation by their spouses in child care. These attitudinal data are consistent with other findings that women whose husbands did actually engage in more child care were less satisfied with their own roles than were women whose husbands participated less (Baruch and Barnett, 1981; cited by Lamb, Pleck, and Levine, 1984).

Further support derives from Russell's (1982) study of role-sharing families in Australia. He found, especially in the early phases of the shift toward shared roles, that there was increased conflict directly associated with the father's increased participation in child care and household tasks. "These conflicts may be due in part to mothers feeling that their traditional domains of housework and child care are threatened when fathers take over these tasks" (Russell and Radin, 1983, p. 150). On the other hand, some (e.g., Bailyn, 1974) reported that women, regardless of their employment status, were more satisfied when their spouses were family-oriented.

In sum, the evidence is inconclusive and further work is necessary to determine explicit measures of mother and father role expectations in mothers and fathers. It is hypothesized that families in which discrepancies between parents are low should be highest in satisfaction. The importance of this issue is underscored by the fact that lack of congruence between roles and beliefs can have negative implications for infants and children. For example, mothers who were working but had strong beliefs about the importance of exclusive maternal care, and nonworking mothers who did not feel that their infants required such care, were most likely to have insecurely attached one-year-olds (Hock, 1978, 1980). These mothers also showed the lowest level of satisfaction with mothering. It is likely that many of these were mothers who were forced to work for financial reasons, or mothers who did not work either because of a feeling of "duty" to mothering or because of the unavailability of suitable infant care or the unwillingness of their spouses to assist. Unfortunately, data concerning the fathers' role in these families were not secured.

INFORMATIONAL SUPPORT

This type of support is available through a variety of sources outside the family, including social-network members, formal agencies, as well as books and periodicals (Clarke-Stewart, 1978). Within the family, the most important predictor of parental competence is the degree of agreement between spouses concerning child-care strategies. Dickie (1984) found that cognitive support, an index of husband-wife agreement about child care, was positively related to maternal and paternal competence. However, as Dickie found in the case of emotional support, cognitive or informational support from the spouse was a more important determinant of fathers' paternal competence. Assessment of the relative importance of intra- in contrast to extrafamilial informational support for the parenting competence of mothers and fathers is a good issue for future research.

The Multiple Nature of Supports

It is convenient for purposes of analysis to discuss each of the types of intrafamilial support separately. Yet we must first recognize that these different types of support interact in natural environments in complex ways and seldom occur singly (Power and Parke, 1984).

Moreover, their impact when occurring alone and in combination with other types of support may, in fact, be different. For example, it is likely that a mother who provides emotional support for her husband does not also offer him informational support and physical assistance.

Second, the nature of the intrafamilial support systems may alter the kinds of extrafamilial supports that family members receive. If the husband gives a great deal of physical support to his wife, she in turn may request it less often from relatives or neighbors; since outside contacts also provide her with social and informational support, she may receive less of those kinds of support as well. It is clear that the interplay among types of support and agents within and outside the family needs to be systematically explored.

Third, the impact of secular changes in employment patterns or childbirth practices on different facets of support needs to be evaluated. Are all types of support equally altered, or do some changes promote greater modifications in some types of support than in others? Similarly, recognition of the diversity of families is important for understanding the impact of secular change on intrafamilial supports. Fathers who respond to their wives' outside employment with a commitment to greater equality in child care may have a different impact than fathers who show no ideological shift.

As families undergo changes, it is critical that we better understand how spouses can assist each other in adjusting to new roles and demands. A family-systems perspective provides a useful framework for this task. By increasing our understanding, we increase our ability to help families adjust successfully to these shifts.

5 *

Single Mothers and
Joint Custody:
Common Ground

A SINGLE MOTHER's struggle for her basic survival and the survival of her children is poignantly captured by Tillie Olsen in a short story, "I Stand Here Ironing." Olsen's narrator discusses the early life of her first child, Emily:

> She was a beautiful baby . . . She was a miracle to me, but when she was 8 months old, I had to leave her daytimes with the woman downstairs to whom she was no miracle at all, for I worked or looked for work and for Emily's father, who "could no longer endure" (he wrote in his goodbye note) "sharing want with us" . . . I was nineteen. It was the pre-relief, pre-WPA world of the Depression. I would start running as soon as I got off the streetcar, running up the stairs, the place smelling sour, and awake or asleep to startle awake, when she saw me she would break into a clogged weeping that could not be comforted, a weeping I can hear yet. (1956, pp. 10–11)

But even as we acknowledge the obvious misery of the child and of the mother who can still hear her weeping, it is the job of professionals to look beneath that emotional pain. For, despite the obvious difficulties, every single-parent household does not disintegrate; not every child in such a household grows up stunted. We must look below the surface of our culture, and there is a lot to see. In 1980, one child in five lived in a single-parent household, a 50 percent increase since 1970 (Children's Defense Fund, 1982). For women between twenty-five and twenty-nine, single-parent births are up 75 percent. Of all births to black women, 50 percent are to single mothers (Weinraub and Wolf, 1983). Of those married in 1977, 49 percent will divorce (Hacker, 1983). Some 40–50 percent of children born in the last decade will spend some years in single parent homes. And 90 percent of those single-parent homes will be headed by women (Hetherington, 1979).

So, as we consider the theme of this book, coping with family stress, we acknowledge that the stresses described by Tillie Olsen are issues of survival. As such, they are our primary consideration. But beneath them lie the mysteries of seemingly random successes and failures in children from fatherless homes. I want to focus on those mysteries here.

In our history of developmental investigations, the nuclear family has remained the sine qua non, providing the optimal framework, we believe, for the emergence of a child's emotional well-being. Different kinds of family organization are often viewed as suboptimal, and single-parent families are thought to be singularly stressful. Weiss (1979), for example, calls the single-parent family "understaffed," because its one-parent head, most often the mother, is forced to assume multiple roles and functions, thereby limiting her parenting capacity. In fact, we have allowed a generation of static group-comparison research to heighten an illusory split, calling dual parenting and dual-parented children "good" and single parenting and the one-parent child "not so good." Such investigations have posited the single parent and the single-parented child to be at greater risk for social and psychic dysfunction when compared to a control group, the married couple and its offspring.

Furthermore, there has been little effort to distinguish between the "state" of single mothering (McClanahan, 1983) and its impact on children, on the one hand, and the stresses related to marital disruption or the absence of fathers (Rutter, 1971), on the other. Then, too, most contemporary research, emphasizing the stress-ridden components of single parenting, has focused primarily on the negative adaptations of the mothers. There has been relatively little written about the single mother's positive adaptations. When we do hear about them, they are usually credited to the absence of demonstrated negative consequences or to the availability of an external support system to "hold things together."

But maternal successes depend on more—in particular, I think, on the mother's inherent parenting strength, on her "internal support system," if you will. What I will look at here I have elsewhere called the mother's capacity for *transitive vitalization* (Atkins, 1981, 1982, 1984a) of the father. Some successful single mothers rely on endogenous psychic strengths to communicate an appropriate, albeit fantasized, "male presence" that facilitates the emotional growth and development of young children. Implicitly, then, I approach the single-mother phenomenon from the perspective of the father's presence or absence.

At the same time, I will consider what seems to be an unfortunate sequel to our frequent disregard of the mother's internal support system: the increasingly frantic legal effort to maintain the illusion of the nuclear family, even when it no longer exists. The fashionable term *joint custody* is often applied to a legislated family "pseudo-nuclearity," which is not always an inevitable or unambiguous advantage in a child's life. A great deal of social policy has been based on what I believe to be two wrong assumptions: that single mothers are always doomed and that joint-custody families are always blessed.

First let us consider the state of single mothering, as influenced by the psychological issues surrounding the absent father. How stressful is a father's absence on the single mother and on her children? The answer is not an easy one, for absent fathering, like single mothering, describes a state for which there are multiple causes and, consequently, disparate stresses. Weinraub and Wolf (1983) have noted that absent fathering affects mothers and children in direct and indirect ways. The direct effects are alleged to be those that result from the "decreased social attention, stimulation, and modeling" provided by the male parent. Indirect effects are those resulting from "increased social, emotional, and financial stresses on the mother" (pp. 1297–98).

Weinraub and Wolf conclude, probably correctly, that the mother's adjustment to these stresses *may* have subsequent effects on the child. But others (Pearlin and Johnson, 1977; Brown and Harris, 1978; Pearlin and Schooler, 1978; Kessler, 1979) have hypothesized, probably incorrectly, that the father's absence *always* exacts a toll on the single mother and her children which is directly proportional to the intensity of the direct and indirect effects of his absence. The indirect factors, in particular, are thought to weigh most heavily. Loss of social supports, reduced financial resources, employment difficulties, problems surrounding child care, and the search for psychic and sexual gratifications (Wallerstein and Kelly, 1980) are all said to contribute to a single mother's diminished parenting effectiveness. It has been suggested that up to 80 percent of divorcing parents leave their children to founder through the emotional vicissitudes of separation, themselves too heavily beset by their own emotional conflicts to provide good parenting (Wallerstein and Kelly, 1975).

Although it goes without saying that these factors may seriously affect the single mother, bad parenting does not necessarily follow. In fact, it may be neither below average nor below expectable. Investigating both single- and two-parent families, Weinraub and Wolf asked whether life changes and available social supports affected the mother's relationship with her children. When families were matched on a number of child, maternal, and income variables, there were no significant differences noticed in mother-child interactions in the two groups. Furthermore, in subdividing mother-child experimental and control group pairs into those with more optimal versus less optimal parent-child interactions, there was an equal distribution of single- and two-parent families in each grouping.

I can confirm these findings on the basis of my own clinical experience. In some single-parent families, the mother's capacity to parent, if good prior to the onset of father absence, might remain fairly good for variable amounts of time following the separation. In other circumstances, seemingly significant stresses imposed by changes in family finances, social supports, and the like have relatively little effect on a single mother's parenting, while other mothers and children experience profound psychic conflict and regression at what might be considered the insignificant "drop of a hat." In still other situations, mothers whose parenting was suboptimal when the father was available become significantly better parents after his departure.

What all but a few investigators fail to take into account, and I believe this is critical, is that the internal worlds of mother and child hold significant, if not exclusive, sway over adaptation to the absent father. First let us consider the mother. Her ability to parent may be affected by external phenomena, but not exclusively. After all, her internal world has been developing throughout her life. Elements that delineate her parenting role include her natural endowment, the growth of her ego structures and functions, especially identifications and object relations, and the reciprocity between her parental initiative and parental responsiveness, on the one hand, and the developmental imperatives of her child and cultural and societal pressures, on the other. These issues have been described by a number of psychoanalytic authors (Anthony and Benedek, 1970; Benedek, 1959 and 1973). Perhaps less studied but equally important to the mother's parenting function involves what I have called her capacity for transitive vitalization of the father and of maleness.

I first became interested in transitive vitalization through my research into the psychic relatedness of very young children to their fathers. This relatedness, it seemed to me, contributed to and was affected by the child's mental representation of his father. Thus I wanted to know something about the emergence of mental registration of each of the parents during infancy.

But the processes that we think are involved in the child's formation of a mental registration of self and object are significantly biased by our current psychoanalytic and cognitive developmental theories. During the last fifty or so years, we have come to believe that the processes of mental registration emerge during the first twelve to eighteen months of life. To oversimplify, we assume that repeated and *direct* sensorimotor contacts with inanimate objects or *direct* reciprocal, drive-mediated transactions with animate objects lead to a series of mental or psychic transformations in the infant. Ultimately, if both inanimate and animate objects are predictable in their behaviors, or to use our catchwords "relatively constant" or "good enough," the child acquires the capacity to image stably, evoke reliably, or represent symbolically such objects, even with no immediate perception. As it pertains to dynamic, available primary-caretaking mothers, this model for the emergence of mental representation may, in fact, seem good enough.

When the scientific observer considers a child's life with the father, however, the model is clearly not good enough. Certainly transactions between father and infant do occur. We have even hypothesized that there are inherent differences between fathers and mothers regarding their "parenting styles" and, consequently, the kind of stimulation that each parent provides an infant or toddler. Yet cross-cultural scrutiny suggests that we cannot be certain that the "aggressive playmate" role we have historically ascribed to fathers always appears as a uniquely paternal phenomenon (Yogman, Parke, Atkins, and Pleck, 1984). Nonetheless, there is a clear discrepancy between our inadvertent wishful idealization of father-infant transactions, particularly as these appear in the psychoanalytic literature, and their actual prevalence. In fact, fathers spend an astonishingly small amount of time with their children. The numbers appear to be too small even to give credence to the homily that quality, not quantity, is what counts in the development of a relationship and its mental representation. To paraphrase from a story by Grace Paley (1978), fatherhood is a Saturday-afternoon profession.

So relative father absence is the developmental norm for very young children, even in typically middle-class nuclear families. But that does not mean that father is a stranger. Because infancy and early toddlerhood are such critical periods in the genesis of representational thinking, I have suggested (1984a) that we reconsider our current ideas about the origin of representational processes, to reincorporate Freud's virtually abandoned notion of drives and drive frustration as an equally important impetus to thinking. Key experiments in the developmental psychology literature which demonstrate that the child verbally labels the father earlier than the mother (Brooks-Gunn and Lewis, 1979) give particular credence to Freud's original propositions.

Although there are limited numbers of father-infant transactions, Parke (1979) and his collaborators have shown that these transactions are significantly affected by the presence of the mother. Parke's work led to my own observation that the mother can indirectly, or transitively, vitalize the father's meaning to his child— she can give the child's "father image" shape and tone, as it were— first in the father's presence and then in his absence. Theoretically I explained the process of transitive vitalization utilizing tenable cognitive and psychoanalytic postulates. Furthermore, in a series of articles, I concluded that the mother's capacity to vivify the father, sometimes larger than life size, or to denigrate and devalue him held clear sway over the child's play about and concomitant representations of the father.

Let me offer a couple of clinical examples from a normal infant nursery which outline the importance of transitive vitalization in the father's absence (Atkins 1981, 1982):

Pete, a rambunctious 2-year-old, loved to engage his mother in many playful activities. One of his special games at the time involved chattering away at his mother in simple sentences. She would chatter back. Often Pete or Mommy could invoke Daddy as a subject of conversation. If, for example, Pete would look inquisitively at Mommy and ask, "Daddy at work?" she would pick up a crayon and paper, start drawing, and say, "Daddy writes at work." She would run wooden cars along the floor: "Daddy drives to work, and then he drives home to see Pete!" Pete, captivated with the activity, joined in her pursuits. One morning in the nursery, while Pete's mother was talking with the other mothers, Pete initiated the play himself. He began, with crayon and paper, to scribble, saying, "Pete work," looking playfully at mother. Mother, having caught sight of the activity in mid-stage, clapped her hands with a delighted chuckle and beamed back at her son. Pete laughed. As the play continued in other contexts, Pete became more engaged in driving the cars himself and in carrying a little doctor's kit, seemingly as a briefcase, around with him. Pete's father representations appeared to blossom, even in the absence of father.

Charlotte, at 23 months, was grossly overweight, as was her mother. The mother, again pregnant and seemingly depressed about it, would come to the nursery because, among other things, it afforded her a social outlet. Charlotte would be plopped on the floor upon arrival, and Mother would pour herself a cup of coffee and pursue conversation with the other adults in the nursery. If, during the nursery time, the other mothers would initiate play with their children, Charlotte's mother would join in. But, she was rarely generative in this regard. Charlotte enjoyed rattling a chain of plastic keys and frequently poked, prodded, and entreated Mother for the rings of house and car keys in her mother's purse. She would pick a key on one or the other ring and twist it on some solid object near Mother. This was frequently accompanied by a somewhat vacuous "Daddy?" and a stare at Mother. If Mother was paying attention, she would respond with a very perfunctory, "Daddy's at work," and then return to her adult conversation. Mother frequently ignored her daughter and refused to provide an answer. Charlotte repeated the question many times during the nursery. Sometimes, when no response was forthcoming, Charlotte would sit and stare for many seconds at the keys she was holding. Although it was impossible to ascertain their exact meaning, the keys seemed to have something to do with Daddy coming home or Daddy going away. Within a short period of time, this play dropped out of the child's repertoire. I saw no additional play about Daddy during the tenure of the nursery, certainly not to the extent that it could be seen with Pete.

It is clear from these examples that the breadth and plasticity of the mother's capacity to parent, influenced by her own inner world, had some, and probably considerable, impact on her child's psychic life with the father.

Now, when we turn to the special circumstance of the single mother, things become somewhat more complicated. It should be clear at this point, though, that my view of father absence in the single-mother situation is not one of phenomenon but rather one of degree.

As with dual-parented youngsters, very young children with no fathers in the home will still construct a father in fantasy, as if now psychically compelled to create what does not exist in fact (Neubauer, 1960). The classic observations of Freud and Burlingham (1943) have shown us that the fantasy formations of children in father-absent families are not a question of phenomenon but, again, one of degree. The circumstances surrounding paternal loss contribute to the affective valence—or emotional tone—associated with the child's father fantasy, often idealizing it positively or negatively. Important to his feeling about his missing father are the timing of the father's loss, the child's developmental phase-specific wishes, and the imperatives imposed by the child's "cultural reality" (Neubauer, 1960).

As part of the child's cultural reality, vicissitudes in the mother's parenting are particularly important. In a time-honored study, Bach (1946) elcited in play the father fantasies of father-separated children, ages six to ten. Fathers of an equivalent distribution of boys and girls had been called into military service when their children were between one and three years old. This group of children was compared to matched controls with fathers at home. In comparison to the control group, the experimental group had, as expected, more positively and negatively idealized fantasies about the absent father. In interviews with the mothers of the children in the experimental group, Bach identified two cohorts possessing different attitudes toward the absent father. In one group, the mothers unambiguously deprecated the absent father; in the other, the mothers were positive and supporting. Among those children who negatively valued the father in fantasy, the mother's attitude toward the father correlated with the degree and intractability of the child's negativity.

In another classic study, Hilgard and Fisk (1960) analyzed optimal adjustment in the children of fatherless families. The most critical factor involved the mother's subsequent parenting strength, particularly her capacity to keep the home intact. She was characterized as strong, responsible, thoughtful, and hard-working. These qualities were thought to engender strong ego development in the affected children, through the mother's serving as a strong but flexible model. She both functioned as an example and fostered or required certain expectations. The strength of the family prior to the father's loss was also important, particularly in those cases where each parent had a well-defined role offering the children "stability and separation tolerance." Once again, the mother's way of talking about her absent husband and her relationship to and attitudes toward men strongly colored her children's feeling about fatherhood, maleness, and their associated representations.

Following Bach's and Hilgard's leads, I want to describe one of my own cases to show some unusual strengths in a single mother, strengths that might not be predicted on the basis of the stresses associated with an absent father. Both her parenting capacities and the ultimately successful psychological adaptation of her child were influenced by her flexible transitive vitalization of the missing father.

Lucine was the single mother of Tyrone, age 8. At 22, Lucine had been in the business of mothering since her own early adolescence. Tyrone was her only child. Tyrone's natural father had never lived in the household, although Lucine moved in with George, three years her senior, shortly after Tyrone was born. They were married when Tyrone was 2½. Lucine had never told Tyrone that George was not his biological father, and Tyrone grew up referring to George as "Dad." George had worked at a series of jobs, most recently in a low white-collar position as a clerk in an insurance company. Lucine worked as a nurse's aide at the local municipal hospital. From the time that Tyrone was a toddler, she had held a stable position on the 4:00 P.M.–12:00 A.M. shift. She was available to Tyrone almost all day during his preschool years. Once school began, Lucine instituted a morning ritual around breakfast for the family. In the afternoon, Lucine would leave for work after her mother arrived to care for Tyrone in the hour or so between her departure for work and George's return home. During the last year, however, Lucine's mother had become ill, and Tyrone had been managing himself at home in the brief after-school period.

In the past six months, Tyrone had been complaining at breakfast that George had been repeatedly late in coming home. While George denied Tyrone's allegations as idle child-hood banter, Lucine decided to surreptitiously stay home one day, calling in sick to her job. When George appeared at home at 9:00 P.M., she confronted him. Quickly she discovered that George was enmeshed in an affair, one of apparently many that she had not known about. She threw him out of the house.

Lucine visited a law clinic in the community to seek a divorce. At the same time, she managed to alter her shift in the hospital to work midnight until 8:00 A.M. With the help of a friendly supervisor, she was able to start work an hour earlier, in order to be home for the breakfast ritual with Tyrone. While she didn't like the fact that she left Tyrone alone overnight, it was the best arrangement she could effect.

Meanwhile, George had taken a new apartment, next to his older sister, Mavis. Apparently furious with Lucine and suffering considerable wounds to his self-esteem, George filed a motion to gain custody of Tyrone. Mavis would care for Tyrone during George's work day. But, legally, the motion made little sense, as George was neither Tyrone's natural father nor had he formally adopted him. But George had failed to reveal these facts to his law clinic attorney.

Lucine could do nothing else but counter George's motion

with the truth about her son's origins. When Tyrone thus discovered the "secret" surrounding his conception, he flew into a rage. For the following two days, he refused to go to school. Lucine became somewhat anxious, felt that she should force him into attendance, but didn't. The next afternoon, following his mother's departure for work, he broke a window in his mother's bedroom with his fist. Removing his bloody hand, he became frightened. He wrapped his hand in his mother's pillowcase and set off, walking two miles, to George's apartment. George immediately took the boy to the municipal hospital emergency room, the same hospital where, five floors above, Lucine was hectically at work. Lucine was brought downstairs to the emergency area to sign the necessary forms for medical treatment. At the same time, she emphatically dismissed George. As he left, Tyrone cried and tried, bloodily, to cling to George's trousers. Lucine called her supervisor, claimed illness, and took her son home. The following morning, Lucine entered Tyrone in the children's mental health clinic.

The psychiatric resident on duty discovered, as a good clinician might, that not only were the events dynamically understandable, but also that the boy's use of his hand was symbolically meaningful. George had, in the weeks prior to the marital dissolution, taught Tyrone how to throw a football. This playtime had become extremely important to Tyrone, as he would admire George's prowess with a ball still much too large for his own childlike hands. Yet Tyrone would also become fiercely competitive, wishing, at least mentally, to best George at his own game. The resident recorded his suspicion that Tyrone's window-breaking episode was, at least in part, reflective of his guilty success at such psychic wishes. When Tyrone rejoined his mother in the waiting room, the resident overheard him tell Lucine, with a brighter disposition than he had managed in some time, "We talked about football!"

With the resident's emphatic support, Lucine accompanied Tyrone to school. That Friday afternoon she returned to work, sensitive to yet mulling the issue of the football. The following morning, while Tyrone was eating breakfast, she changed into a sweatsuit, rarely worn, and returned to the kitchen with Tyrone's football. Her exhaustion notwithstanding, she took to the streets with her clearly ambivalent son. Now, Lucine knew nothing about football, understood her limitations, but attempted a pass. The ball, naturally, lobbed erratically for a few feet. Tyrone stared at his bandaged hand, refusing to look at the mess his mother had made. Lucine retrieved the football and tried again. Still Tyrone looked at the ground. Finally, she picked up the ball and went to her disgruntled son.

"Look," she said, "I'm a girl. I don't know anything about this stuff." Tyrone picked up the ball and, cradling it in his mitten-like bandage, pierced the air for a few feet. Lucine tried to catch the ball but failed. "Damn," she said, "we girls just *don't have what it takes*! You've got it, Tyrone. You do it like a boy!" Tyrone protested, loudly voicing the limitations of his bandaged hand. "It doesn't matter," Lucine countered. "Even with that, it's *more than I've got* with this ball! Soon you'll be as good as George, better probably!"

The psychiatric resident continued to meet with Tyrone during the next two months. Saturday morning football had become a ritual between mother and son. It was quite clear that Lucine had, rather sensitively but not necessarily consciously, provided Tyrone with a thinly veiled but sublimated outlet for his incestuous wishes, permission for "outdoing George," while also clearly fostering or transitively facilitating an appropriate sense of maleness and masculinity in the youngster. She managed to keep the divorce proceedings between herself and George, without unnecessarily involving Tyrone.

Follow-up four months later revealed Tyrone doing well at school with no apparent evidence of ongoing psychic dysfunction.

In a fictional, but related, context Grace Paley describes a single mother, Faith, accomplishing the same task with her two sons. Faith declares:

"You're an American child. Free. Independent." Now what does that mean? I have always required a man to be dependent on, even when it appeared that I had one already. I own two small boys whose dependence on me takes up my lumpen time and my bourgeois feelings. I'm not the least bit ashamed to say that I tie their shoes and I have wiped their backsides well beyond the recommendations of my friends, Ellen and George Hellsbraun, who are psychiatric social workers and appalled. I kiss those kids forty times a day. I punch them *just like a father should.*   (1978, p. 229; italics added)

Of course, there was more to Tyrone's successful adjustment than a football. His mother and Grace Paley's Faith were able to create an illusory sense of the father's vitality, even though their sons no longer had the same kind of contact with them. The fear that such successes are rare, however, has created an ironic alternative—one that I believe may generate as much or more stress than it tries to ease. In their wish to continue the integrity of dual parenting, or at least to preserve its outlines, those who generate social policy and legal decisions for the children of divorce have invented, or at least given preference to, joint custody. As the custodial disposition of over one million children a year (Steinman, 1981) makes the problem epidemic in proportion, some well-known and respected family therapists, among them Roman and Haddad (1978) and Greif (1979), have argued that only joint custody serves the best interests of all affected children. The emotional climate is such that in some states, California, Oregon, Iowa, and Wisconsin among them, joint custody has become the legally mandated custodial disposition for the children of divorce. Thirty states currently have some form of joint-custody law; in every remaining state, such a law is pending.

Joint custody is the aggregate of three characteristics that distinguish it from sole custody (Benedek and Benedek, 1979). First, both parents are required to assume equal responsibility for the physical, emotional, and moral development of their children. Second, parents must share the rights and responsibilities for making decisions that affect their children. (These two points define joint legal custody of the affected children.) Third, there must be joint physical custody: the child is supposed to live with each parent for a substantial period of time.

Proponents of joint custody have argued that it accomplishes two aims: it distributes the frequency of interaction more evenly between the child and each parent, and it increases the frequency of interaction and cooperation between divorced parents on child-related issues. I think there is no evidence to suggest that such a legal mandate is desirable, or that a joint disposition inevitably works better than sole custody in fostering a child's emotional and social development (Atkins, 1984b).

From my analysis of recent contributions outlining positive and negative post-divorce outcomes in parents and children, it seems clear that the number of contacts children have with their non-custodial father is relevant only if such contacts are reasonably pleasurable. In the absence of definable mental illness in either children or parents, the positive experience of noncustodial contact correlates with positive post-divorce adaptation in the parents, particularly related to diminishing amounts of interparent acrimony.

Finally, if one looks at the persistence of interparent anger or animosity, leading to negative experiences for the children of divorce, one finds essentially the same statistics among both sole-custody and joint-custody children. In different samples, approximately one quarter to one third of parents in either group continue to make it difficult for their children to adapt. Of those children who do adapt well, there appear to be virtually no differences between those in sole custody and those in joint custody over time.

In the one quarter to one third of vulnerable families in either group, what does continuing parental conflict cost the child? Does it, in fact, inhibit what Lucine was able to build alone? In clinical work with the children and parents of divorce, Bernstein and Robey (1962) noted the need for "exposing and controlling the hostility of divorced parents . . . in order to avoid the many ways in which this anger [can] disrupt the child's development." Derdeyn (1983) suggested that clinical work with children and parents after divorce centers on "adults who are angry if not also depressed and children who are depressed if not also overtly angry. This describes a situation where neither parents nor children can be very rewarding to each other" (p. 386).

Derdeyn describes how parental anger can act as a contagion in the emotional lives of children. Putting his mechanisms primarily in descriptive terms, he suggests that parental anger will have "a corrosive effect on a child's sense of security and self-esteem." A further, more specific problem arises when "a parent's anger, rooted in narcissistic injury and abandonment by the other parent, comes to involve the children as stand-ins or messengers of that other parent" (p. 387). In the half dozen or so clinical examples that Derdeyn gives, he does not elaborate how many children are in sole or joint custody. But, based on statistical observations, we can safely assume that most of Derdeyn's children are in sole custody.

Let me illustrate, from my clinical experience, some of the ways that parental conflict manifests itself in the emotional disequilibrium of the children of joint custody. Throughout this exposition, you will doubtless hear the echo of Derdeyn's observations, elaborated in a somewhat more psychoanalytic context. As a first and perhaps obvious example, parental discord can intersect with a child's developmental needs:

> Evan, at 6½, was an overtly oedipal child when he was initially brought to see me, manifestly preoccupied with his strength, independence and functional capacities. His parents' joint custody was legally implemented in the month prior to his first consultation. Evan spent four days a week at his mother's apartment, which had been the only home he had known, and three days a week at his father's apartment. Evan, an only child, began to have bad dreams shortly after his father left, usually involving "dizzy dancing" with a "lady in a dress." The thinly veiled sexual nightmare seemed to characterize both his wish and fear to be alone in the house with mother. During the remainder of the week, he would rather blandly troop to his father's apartment, convinced that, while he was with father, mother was busy having a baby. Once the baby arrived, Evan would be rejected and discarded, just as he felt his father had been. As a consequence of the intersection of his developmental dilemma and his living arrangements, Evan spent four days a week hyperexcited and three days a week depressed. When I mentioned to the parents that they be a bit less compulsive about the alternating physical custody, the mother agreed—even to the point of suggesting that the child live for a time with father until he "settled down." Father would not hear of it, and he imposed his own rejection. He argued that any changes in the living arrangement violated the spirit of joint custody, which he "had paid dear money to obtain."

As with sole-custody parents, joint-custody parents are not exempted from neurotic attempts to repeat and to work through libidinally or aggressively tinged conflicts with their former spouses. Often these conflicts are partially displaced onto the child, or the child is incorporated into the parents' neurotic behaviors. Invariably these behaviors will either negatively affect a child's developmental requirements or will induce a regression as the child attempts to rework a prior conflict. For example:

Mrs. Greenberg brought 9-year-old Justin to see me because
the boy "had trouble expressing his feelings." The mother put
great stock in the expression of *her* feelings, almost to the point
of vomiting them out. She had entered therapy some months
before, in order to "get some things off my chest" at the time
her divorce had become final. Manifestly the mother professed
her love for Justin and his 6-year-old sister. But a reaction-
formation was quite clear. She gave the impression that if her
love were not eagerly incorporated by her children, she would,
with determination, shove it into any available orifice. Justin
was terrified of his mother, cowering in a corner of the room,
never taking his eyes off this incessantly talkative woman. Mrs.
Greenberg proudly claimed that she had engineered a joint-
custody arrangement with Justin's father, a milquetoast per-
sonified. According to the arrangement, Justin and his sister
spent three nights a week in the father's studio apartment,
sleeping on a sofa bed, while the father was forced to sleep
on the floor. While the father thought, during the custody
hearing, that joint custody would allow him some preservation
of masculinity, he also might have known his wife better than
that. At the time I saw Justin, neither the boy nor his father
wanted the nights at father's home. But mother steadfastly
insisted. Ostensibly, she wanted her "freedom to go out with
the girls." Latently, she enjoyed forcing Justin into repeated
participation in her ongoing castration of the father. In one
early session, Justin announced that his favorite story was Hansel and Gretel, "especially the part where Hansel pushes the
witch into the oven."

Some joint-custody parents continue to battle with one another
in a fascinating way. Manifestly, these parents are in complete
support of joint custody and its requirements. But subtly they
undermine it, using what they believe its requirements to be in the
service of their continuing war with one another. Let me elaborate:

Alicia was a somewhat plump, buck-toothed, blonde 12-
year-old when she first came to me for consultation. Her parents had been divorced ten months before. Her father lived
in Connecticut, and her mother, soon to be remarried, lived
just across the New York border in Westchester County. Alicia
spent alternating weeks with her father and mother. She went
to school in Westchester, at a private coeducational day school.

The school was about equidistant from each parent's home. During one week, Alicia would board the schoolbus in her mother's community; in the next week she'd use the bus in her father's. Father was a well-to-do attorney. It was he who, when the marriage was on the rocks, suggested joint custody. Mother, a psychiatrist, was initially reluctant, but, after she consumed the then-available literature on the subject of joint custody, acquiesced.

Initially, Alicia looked depressed, although she had a hard time verbalizing her sadness. A pervasive worry, almost an obsession, began to fill the early hours: "What," she wondered, "was a lesbian?" Could some woman love other women to the exclusion of men? As we began to talk, Alicia revealed a striking anxiety about men. She couldn't even think about them without looking like a wreck.

In the fourth week of our twice-weekly sessions, we had an unusual Saturday morning appointment. I work on Saturday for a couple of hours, but Alicia had never before been to my office on that day of the week. During the rest of the week I wear a jacket and tie in the office—on Saturdays I dress more casually. On that particular Saturday I wore a pair of running shoes, which she noticed immediately.

"Adidas," she noted, then giggled. "What's funny?" I asked.

"You know what it stands for?" she inquired. "No," I said.

"A-D-I-D-A-S," she spelled. "All I Do Is Dream About Sex!" She smiled. "Do you?" I inquired.

She looked at the floor and nodded while pursing her lips. The dreams began a few months before, shortly after she had gotten an ambivalently longed-for dog. They were of nightmarish intensity, and clearly graphic representations of herself about to engage in some kind of thinly veiled sexual activity. She would always wake up before she saw the person with whom she was involved. At first she insisted, rather vehemently, that her partner must be a woman—hence her homosexual "anxiety." But quickly she associated to men, dropping the apparently regressive defense. Her anxiety began to mount. She told me that she didn't like being unable to see the other person in the dream. When I asked what she thought about it, she blurted out: "Well, then, it could be anybody! I mean someone ridiculous—like my father even!" The truth was out.

In subsequent sessions, I asked more about the acquisition of the dog. Alicia thought she had wanted a dog for as long as she could remember. As she talked about it, the dog was at one and the same time a playmate, a sibling, a toy, and, most important, her baby. When her parents were married, mother adamantly refused to consider having a dog in the home. Mother had assumed, probably correctly, that the responsibility for its care would fall to her, and this dual-career family simply did not need additional dependent entities. Father, during the marriage, seemed more open to the idea of a dog. The dog became an area for conspiracy between Alicia and her father. They would occasionally talk about how they would get one together, if only mother weren't in the way. In the end, however, father acquiesced to his wife's reluctance. For Alicia, while her parents were married, the dog symbolized something to wish for—but not to have. She had been content with that working through of the situation. I'll return to the dog shortly.

In a meeting with me, mother described the demise of the marriage. This fifteen-year "fiasco," as she called it, was doomed from its first year, when sex between the spouses all but dried up. Her rather obsessional lawyer-husband just seemed to lose interest, investing his sexual energies into the collection of the erotic sculptures which had populated their living room. Mother delighted in telling me how, when father left, "those damned pricks left with him." There was not much doubt about her feeling or her problem.

The two of them would fight constantly. Inevitably, father's obsessional "legal eagle" shrewdness would hold sway. He would mentally outmaneuver his wife. Occasionally, these mind games were totally irrational. Despite her significant intellect and her psychiatric training, mother would play nonetheless. Once she referred to the man as a "mind fucker." At that point I told her she had traded sex for getting screwed in other, perhaps more tolerable, ways.

When it was clear that a divorce was imminent, and when father sold mother the idea of joint custody, the outward content of their relationship changed. They stopped arguing. Both parents agreed, or thought they did, that the bickering must end "in order to provide Alicia with all that she would need during this period of stress." They agreed to have bi-weekly, then once-monthly, meetings with each other to discuss Alicia's welfare—and to try to keep their split parenting consistent. What probably transpired at these meetings was latently much more loaded, as the episodes surrounding the dog will exemplify.

They sold their home, and each parent moved into smaller quarters. When mother finally moved to Westchester, she raised the issue of Alicia's schooling at one of the meetings with her ex-husband. It was perfectly reasonable that Alicia attend the school in Westchester which mother had chosen. But father saw room to maneuver. He fabricated having visited a girls' school near his new home in Connecticut and suggested that mother, Alicia, and he visit the facility to see if the girl would like it better than the Westchester academy. Mother didn't call the bluff. Instead she did what she had always done. She began to worry. As she had done in the marriage, she began to look for other things to "give in to" in order to protect her daughter's education. It was a rehash of the marital situation. Mother wanted to trade a big screwing for little ones. Father suggested that he would retreat from the school issue if mother would give in to the dog. Somehow, father argued, the dog and Alicia would be transported each week between the two homes. Although mother claimed, rightly, that Alicia had not brought the subject of a dog to light in recent months, she nonetheless capitulated almost instantly.

Unfortunately, to Alicia, this new attitude toward dogs was just too gratifying. The old family saw, wherein some things, like dogs, were not to be had no matter how much you wished, was exchanged for a new religion wherein anything was possible. Significant oedipal reactivation, with fulminating conflicts surrounding drive and defense, was being worked out on the developmental eve of her adolescence. The timing, it seemed to me, was less than perfect.

Then, too, I think Alicia knew that. One day when she didn't feel much like talking in the session, she found her way to crayons and paper. She drew a rabbit, staring straight out of the paper, with Alicia-like buck teeth in its mouth. A rainbow encased the animal peacefully on the paper. But on either side of the rainbow, she portrayed a veritable deluge. She and I knew that she was wishing for some solace from the torrents of her intrapsychic conflicts.

Would things have been the same or different in this family, and especially for the child, if there had been sole custody with the mother? Could Alicia's mother have organized her parenting as Lucine did for Tyrone? It is hard to tell. But it is clear that the unique vicissitudes of joint custody imposed their rather massive horns upon this girl's sizeable dilemma.

Just what have these unhappy children shown us? Whatever is going on in their lives, things are probably not as good as they could be. In each case, the joint-custody arrangement appears to be just another weapon in a vicious parental arsenal: spouse versus spouse. It increases stress on the child as well.

As I have stated, this does not mean that joint custody is always bad. But to have it legislated as the first option for judges and parents—when the marital pathology often guarantees that the shared child will become a shared weapon—is a presumption that violates the purpose of all custodial deliberations: the best interests of the child. As in all other human endeavors, human nature is not among those things that can be legislated. What looks good on the outside depends too much upon what is happening on the inside.

To conclude, in both single-parent situations and joint-custody families, I believe that professionals have had their so-called scientific attitude shaped by misperceptions and prejudices often based on cliché. We have turned our heads toward single-mother families and have seen a vessel half empty, a family drained of a father's availability and weakened by the alleged stresses imposed on family stability and the single mother's functioning. We rarely notice the single mother's successful adaptations, struggles though these may be. There are doubtless many pathways to such adaptations: transitive vitalization may be one of them. Defining these pathways is a real challenge, for they remain poorly delineated and inadequately studied (Leahey, 1984).

In the case of joint custody, we have taken this supposedly half-empty vessel and filled it with great expectations. As Derdeyn and Scott (1984) note, "there is a marked disparity between the power of the joint custody movement and the sufficiency of evidence that joint custody can accomplish what we expect of it" (p. 207). If children's welfare is our business, and the best interests of children are on our minds, we must take care to draw sufficiently upon lessons of strength wherever we find them—neither insisting on weakness where there is none nor fabricating facile solutions when problems are far too complex—and we must find the ways to pass along, for the sake of the children, the lessons we learn.

III *

Forces Outside
the Family:
Work and Family Life

＊ _____

B y EXPLORING the relation between work and family life, this third part illustrates the links among the family system, the work environment, and child care. The workplace has failed to adjust to dramatic changes in family structure. Most jobs are still set up as if the typical family were composed of a man who goes out to work and leaves his wife home with the children, even though less than 10 percent of families in the United States now fit this model. Recently, a Family Policy Panel of the United Nations Association of the United States (*New York Times*, January 7, 1986), composed of corporate executives, union presidents, academics, and former President Gerald Ford, recommended paid leave for women, unpaid leave for men, and government and business involvement in ensuring high-quality child care and flexible work schedules. In view of the fact that most industrialized nations have family-leave policies, these recommendations were seen as an investment in this nation's future.

When one examines the linkages between the family and the workplace, certain constructs from systems theory, such as the degree of communication and feedback between working parents and their workplace managers, help to explain the degree of difficulty in integrating the two spheres. If managers do not pay attention to the needs of their working parents, the workplace is likely to receive such negative outcomes as decreased productivity. Analyses of excellence and high productivity in America's best-run companies find open and responsive management styles to be characteristic.

Each chapter in this section examines these issues from a different perspective. Ann Crouter and Maureen Perry-Jenkins provide a historical look at studies of parental employment and argue strongly for a systems concept of the link between the effects of employment on parents and on children. They point out the advantages of examining the impact of stresses and supports in the workplace on the entire family system, as opposed to earlier studies of maternal employment and child development. Ellen Galinsky reports on attempts within the corporate sector to develop innovative programs that support workers and their families, particularly if they are likely to enhance productivity. Abraham Zaleznik examines work-family conflicts from an intrapersonal, psychodynamic perspective. He contrasts the values and defenses used by managers to succeed at work with those that are adaptive in a family environment. Finally, the chapter by Gwen Morgan on supplemental child care is included in this part because of the close connection between the need for good child care and the widespread phenomenon of two working parents.

ANN C. CROUTER and
MAUREEN PERRY-JENKINS

6 ✳

Working It Out: Effects of Work on Parents and Children

Sigmund Freud is said to have defined maturity in adulthood as the capacity to love and to work. Recent research confirms the importance of these phenomena in most people's lives (Smelser, 1980). A number of surveys have revealed the centrality of close, loving relationships—particularly family relationships—for adults (Berscheid and Peplau, 1983). Moreover, studies of unemployment depicting the often devastating impact of job loss on individuals and families are evidence of the role that work plays in people's lives. Our goal in this chapter is to discuss one aspect of the interrelationship between love and work by summarizing research on the ways in which parents' work situations affect relationships within the family, specifically the marital relationship and parent-child relationships.

Parental work situations represent both stresses and supports for parents and children, depending upon a host of circumstances. Some of these circumstances include whose job it is—the mother's or the father's—how satisfied the individual is with the job, how much time is involved, how the family manages tasks such as housework and supervising children, and characteristics of the children involved, including age, gender, and temperament. In this chapter we attempt to organize this complex set of research findings to convey a sense of how important both the family's position in the larger social environment and the family's internal dynamics are to understanding how parents' work roles affect family members.

Several themes will emerge in our discussion. First, studies on the effects of parents' work mirror the historical times in which they were carried out (Bronfenbrenner and Crouter, 1982). For example, research conducted prior to 1960 on how mothers' employment affected children reflected the zeitgeist of the time. These studies looked for negative effects—and found them.

Second, researchers have asked very different questions about the employment of men versus that of women (Kanter, 1977). The assumption for years was that women who work outside the home were a social problem, a threat to marital harmony and optimal child development. Similarly, it was held that unemployment for husbands and fathers was a social problem with grave consequences for the family. As society's notions about the appropriate roles for men and women have changed, researchers have slowly begun to ask new questions.

A third and related issue is that there is growing recognition that the family is a system. This perspective implies that we should be interested in the *processes* that link the family to the workplaces of its breadwinners. In addition, we should be prepared to examine how, for example, the quality of a couple's marriage buffers the child from the potentially negative consequences of stressful work conditions. Similarly, this perspective alerts us to the importance of phenomena outside the immediate family context, including emotional support provided by friends and kin, the availability of high-quality child care, and the changing nature of the economy within which parents' jobs are imbedded.

A Systems Perspective on Work-Family Issues

First and foremost, many families with young children today are dual-earner families. Thus studies of two-parent families need to consider the contributions of both parents' jobs. All too often, researchers focus on the fact that mother works (or doesn't work) and ignore the role that father's job may play in the family. For example, how smoothly do the parents' work schedules mesh? How are husband and wife dividing the housework? How supportive is each partner of the other spouse's commitment both to work and to family life?

A second issue is that young children in dual-earner families usually spend a large portion of the day in some form of child care. It is therefore unfortunate that separate studies have been conducted on the impact of daycare and the effects of having two working parents, limiting our ability to see what families are experiencing as they balance work, family, and child-care arrangements.

A third issue to keep in mind is that we know from other research that children are affected by the quality of their parents' marriage (see Belsky, 1981). Thus we should examine how the parents' marital relationship either buffers the child from possible work-related stresses or fails to do so, a perspective that views family relationships as an intricate, interrelated system.

Finally, children may affect their parents in ways that shape how the parent responds to his or her job. A healthy, happy child may serve as an affirmation that the parent is doing a good job, at work and at home. A parent with an unhappy child—a child who acts out, fails to do well in school, or cannot make friends—may have more doubts about how well he or she is balancing work and family responsibilities. Similarly, studies of the effects of employment on the marital relationship often ignore the possibility that the child's response may influence the parents' reactions. In fact, these studies usually ignore the presence of children completely. Recognition that children and parents reciprocally influence each other's development is a hallmark of the systems perspective.

One Couple's Experiences

Before describing research on the influence of employment on the family, it may be useful to offer an illustration of a couple struggling with the issue of how to coordinate two work roles and a fulfilling marital relationship. Mary and Michael Perkins are a couple who have recently participated in the Penn State Pair Project (Huston, McHale, and Crouter, in press), a longitudinal study of the development of conjugal relations over the first two years of married life. One of the goals of the pair project was to examine the role that the work situations of husbands and wives play in influencing their relationship. We know quite a lot about Mary and Michael's work and family lives through information drawn from structured questionnaires, telephone interviews, and open-ended interviews.

Mary and Michael Perkins were married in 1981 and have both been employed full-time ever since. Throughout the study, Michael has been employed as a bank accountant and works about forty hours a week. Mary was a schoolteacher during the time of her first interview, two months after her marriage. She subsequently made a career shift and became a computer operator. Her new line of work is more lucrative than teaching but has other costs, as Mary is the first to note. At the time of her second interview, about a year after marriage, Mary was working as much as sixty hours a week due to a personnel shortage at her firm. The couple's work schedules were usually quite similar, beginning work about 8:30 and leaving at 4:30 in the afternoon. During the personnel shortage, however, Mary routinely worked from 8:30 A.M. to 8:30 P.M.

Mary and Michael differ in terms of how much they like their jobs. Despite the long hours, Mary rates her job as highly satisfying. She has received several pay raises in quick succession and feels good about what she is doing. Michael is less satisfied. The work itself has become routine and unchallenging, and he expressed discontent in his last two interviews with the rate of his progress within the organization.

One of the most obvious advantages of the Perkins' lifestyle is two paychecks. During their second interview, Michael commented, "My wife and I have set some goals as far as purchasing a house by this summer. We sat down and budgeted ourselves to allow us to live off my wife's paycheck and bank mine . . . We're both very happy about our financial situation."

At the time of the last interview, which took place approximately two years after their marriage, Mary and Michael had bought that house. Both were continuing to pursue their career goals. Moreover, Mary was pregnant. Both spouses wondered how they would manage to get everything done when a baby was added to their already busy lives. They sought reassurance from their interviewers that the child's development would not be in jeopardy because of their dual-earner lifestyle. When describing what research has been done on the impact of husbands' and wives' work on the family, we will refer back to Mary and Michael Perkins and provide illustrations from their interviews that exemplify important themes in the literature in this area.

Our organizational strategy is to begin by discussing work's impact on the marital relationship and then subsequently to explore its effects on children. Within these two sections, we attempt to convey how the development of knowledge has evolved across historical time and how research frequently mirrors society's changing ideas about what men and women should be doing. Because they are invariably studied separately, within each section we will first discuss women and their work, then men and theirs.

Consequences for the Marital Relationship

WIVES' EMPLOYMENT

Early research on the impact of wives' employment on the marriage relationship frequently assumed that the wife's decision to work would have detrimental consequences. Couples would be less satisfied with their relationship; the power dynamic would be disrupted; and housework would become an arena of conflict. The working wife was an emotional issue for scholars of the time. The contemporary reader of one of the first essays on the topic, which appeared in the *American Journal of Sociology* in 1909, is struck by the emotionally charged language of the piece:

> The proportion of sober and steady men is nearly twice as great in families where the wives do not work as in homes presided over by employed wives. While it cannot, of course, be assumed that all delinquent husbands have been demoralized by abnormal home conditions, the conviction of such causal relation is the natural and logical one. (Weatherly, 1909, p. 745)

Despite the common assumption that employed wives represented a threat to marital bliss, studies that actually tested this hypothesis found that the relationship was more complex. A 1949 study by Locke and Mackeprang compared the marital adjustment of women in full-time employment versus full-time homemaking and found no differences. In addition, the husbands of these two groups of wives did not differ in their marital adjustment. A subsequent investigation (Gianopulos and Mitchell, 1957) concluded that the husband's attitude about his wife's decision to work was a critical factor. The spouses reported greater conflict (especially about housework and childrearing) if the wife worked *and* the husband disapproved of her working, as opposed to if she worked and her husband approved or if she did not work outside the home. Other studies (Rivers, Barnett, and Baruch, 1979) concur that marital satisfaction is enhanced when spouses share a clear agreement about who in the family should work outside the home.

All work situations are not alike, however. One critical issue is how satisfied the woman is with her job. Wives who enjoy their jobs tend to be more satisfied with married life than those who do not enjoy their work (Nye, 1959). Moreover, there are social-class differences in this regard. In working-class families, homemakers tend to be more satisfied with their marriages than women employed full time. Why? The job opportunities open to working-class women are limited and tend to be unsatisfying. In addition, a working-class woman who can afford to stay home usually is married to a man who is a successful breadwinner, an important element of marital happiness, particularly for women with traditional values.

Since about 1960, the issue of marital power has been a major focus of attention in research on the employment of wives (see the review by Huston, 1983). These studies document that not only does the employed wife have more power in family decision making but that her influence increases as her income and job prestige increase relative to her husband's. This consistent finding has been explained using resource theory that assumes that marital power is determined in large part by the resources each partner brings to the relationship. Earnings and independence acquired on the job give the wife enhanced bargaining power at home.

If the employed wife acquires power in family decision making, is she able to bargain for a more equitable division of household tasks? A comment by Michael Perkins, the husband in our case study above, suggests that this might be true. Asked to describe how he felt about the way he and Mary divided housework, he replied,

At first I was probably dissatisfied just because I wasn't used to doing that sort of work, like running around doing the vacuuming or doing the dusting—I just wasn't used to doing it and I thought, Gee, this shouldn't be my job. This isn't my part. But I came to learn that my wife holds down a full-time job also and she shouldn't be responsible for all the household tasks. It wasn't fair.

Early research suggested that when wives were employed outside the home, their husbands did do more work around the house (Blood and Wolfe, 1960). But these studies relied on proportional measures of family work, meaning that husbands with employed wives performed a greater percentage of the housework accomplished. In the mid-1960s and early 1970s, several investigations focused on the actual amount of time spent on housework. Walker and Woods (1976), for example, found that in families in which the wife was a homemaker, she spent about 8.1 hours per day on housework, while her husband spent 1.6 hours per day. When the wife was employed full time, her time in housework dropped to 4.8 hours per day. Her husband put in . . . 1.6 hours. Is it any wonder that the wife in a dual-earner marriage has been described as suffering from "role overload" (Rapoport and Rapoport, 1976)?

Recent analyses suggest that men are increasing their involvement in housework (Pleck, 1983), but progress is slow. Interestingly, men seem to be increasing their participation *regardless* of whether or not their wives hold full-time jobs, presumably because our norms about the role of husband and father appear to be gradually shifting in the direction of greater involvement in family life.

To our knowledge, virtually no research has focused on the impact of the wife's work *schedule* on marriage, although there have been studies of this kind with regard to men's jobs, as will be discussed later. It is likely that the number of hours the wife spends at work and the timing of those hours in relation to her husband's workday influences how much time they can spend together. This was a major theme in Michael and Mary's second interview, during the time when Mary was working sixty hours a week on a routine basis. Mary explained that they rarely had time to relax together on weekdays and that they disagreed about how to spend time on weekends. Exhausted from a long week, Mary wanted to sleep and relax on the weekend, while Michael looked forward to socializing with friends and doing leisure activities together as a couple. These differences in their needs produced conflicts that Mary and Michael had to work through. They expressed great relief when Mary's work schedule returned to normal.

HUSBANDS' EMPLOYMENT

What is known about the impact of the husband's job on his relationship with his wife? Not surprisingly, given social norms about the appropriate roles for men and women, researchers have asked different questions about men's employment than they have about women's. It is difficult to find studies on the impact of husband's employment on marital satisfaction or the effects of his job on his involvement in housework because it has been assumed that a husband's place is in the labor force. Instead, a husband's unemployment has been the social problem to interest researchers. For years, a husband's work situation was a family issue only when it was missing.

From studies conducted during the Great Depression to recent studies on plant closings, there is much evidence that a husband's unemployment often puts a strain on the marital adjustment and satisfaction of both partners. The combination of the loss of identity provided by work and the tendency for the unemployed husband to spend more and more time at home can result in disrupted family routines and new strains and tensions. As with wives' employment, the impact of the husband's unemployment seems to depend upon a variety of factors. Voydanoff (1983) summarizes these factors under two headings: (1) the family's definition of the situation; (2) the family's resources. By "definition of the situation," Voydanoff refers to the fact that marriages are differentially affected by husband's unemployment depending upon how sudden the event is, the extent to which the wife sees the loss of the job as her husband's fault, and the extent to which she perceives him to be failing in his role as breadwinner. Similarly, resources such as a financial cushion, social support from kin and friends, and the strength of the marital bond before the loss of the job influence how the marriage will fare.

Not surprisingly, when husbands experience unemployment, the balance of power often shifts in the wife's direction, particularly if she enters the labor force at this time (Elder, 1974; Komarovsky, 1940). Husbands experiencing unemployment do not usually throw themselves enthusiastically into housework, but it is likely that when they do *not* participate in household tasks, tension and strains increase.

There is much more involved with a husband's job than simply employment status. Indeed, almost fifty years ago, sociologist Willard Waller recognized the importance of the husband's work situation to the marriage when he wrote in his well-known monograph on the family:

> The economic situation of the family affects the conflict processes within it profoundly. The long arm of the job reaches into the home and sets husband and wife against one another. Occupations which have high contact mobility have correspondingly high divorce rates. The person who considers himself a failure in his occupation is likely to compensate by becoming a domestic tyrant . . . Nor must we neglect to mention those families wrecked by success.   (1938, pp. 335–336)

More recently, some empirical research evidence has emerged to support the assumption that the nature of the work that husbands do affects their marital relationship. For example, a 1981 study by Burke and Weir found that job stresses such as work overload, responsibility for other workers, job ambiguity, and job complexity were all negatively associated with marital satisfaction. This seems to vary depending upon the personality of the man involved. Men with Type A personalities—people described as competitive, aggressive, restless, and driven—seem to be especially at risk to bring work stress home. In some of our own research, we have found that the more husbands report feeling stressed and tired at the end of the workday, the less likely they are to do housework and the more likely they are to engage in negative interactions (such as criticizing or complaining) with their wives (Crouter, Perry-Jenkins, and Huston, in preparation).

The timing of the work that men do makes a mark on their relationships with their wives. Mott, Mann, McLoughlin, and Warwick (1965) explored the impact of working different shifts on men's family relationships. They concluded that the night shift, traditionally beginning at 11:00 P.M. and ending at 7:00 A.M., interferes with employees' marital relationships. Not surprisingly, their respondents cited sexual relations as one of the aspects of marriage to be most disrupted by working the night shift.

To summarize some of the key points made so far, work and marriage are clearly not separate worlds. Not only does the employment status of husband and wife make a difference, but factors such as how satisfied they are with their jobs, how each partner views the other partner's work situation, and how much income and occupational prestige are derived from the job are just a few of the conditions that help to shape work's impact on the marital relationship. In addition, researchers have not been blind to cultural stereotypes about the roles of men and women, a theme that will be even more pronounced in the next domain we want to explore: the impact of parents' work on their children.

Consequences for Children

It may seem odd that we discuss the marriage relationship and parent-child relations separately. After all, isn't the family a system? Shouldn't the impact of parents' work on children depend in part on how the husband and wife handle it between themselves? Obviously, it would be preferable to present an integrated picture of the familial consequences of parental employment. But, to a great extent, such a picture does not emerge in the literature. Thanks in part to the specialization of foci within the social sciences, family sociologists have tended to study work's impact on marriage while developmental psychologists have focused on the impact of work (usually mother's work) on the child. We are a long way from understanding the complexities of the dual-earner family as a system.

MATERNAL EMPLOYMENT

In a recent review, Bronfenbrenner and Crouter (1982) note that, prior to about 1960, scholars were virtually unanimous in their assessment that maternal employment had negative consequences for children. In 1909, for example, Weatherly noted, "It is in relation to childhood that the disorganizing effects of female labor are most discernible" (p. 745).

Most of Weatherly's ideas were not grounded in solid research findings. Rather, they reflected views that were widely held at the time. Early empirical studies emphasized negative outcomes for children, such as maladjustment and delinquency. These studies had major methodological flaws, however, including a tendency to confound maternal employment and social class. By the end of the 1950s, when studies were better designed, it appeared that having a mother in the labor force was not related to delinquency, adolescent maladjustment, poor school grades, or dependency behavior in kindergarteners.

Since about 1960, there has been an explosion of research on the impact on children of having a mother in the labor force. So much has been done that it would be impossible to review it all in a brief chapter. Instead we focus on some of the more interesting findings. One of the heartening trends in this research is an increased tendency to try to identify family processes that take place in families with employed mothers versus those with full-time homemaker mothers.

A common question and one that concerned Mary and Michael Perkins is, "Do infants whose mothers are in the paid labor force have more difficulty forming attachments to their mothers than infants whose mothers are homemakers?" Although early research suggested that this might be true, recent research indicates that this is not usually a problem. One reason may be that babies with working mothers have been found to receive as much one-to-one interaction as their counterparts whose mothers are homemakers (Goldberg, 1977). At least in middle-class homes, mothers seem to be able to structure their schedules so that they spend a sufficient amount of time with their infants. Not enough research has been done in working-class families, however, to know whether families with fewer resources manage as successfully. In addition, much of this research has been done on firstborn children. Mothers with jobs may have difficulty spending time with their babies if older children are competing for their attention.

Another issue of concern to working parents is, "How will having an employed mother affect my child's performance in school?" Prior to 1960, researchers would probably have predicted negative outcomes for school-aged children of employed mothers. Recent studies portray a more complex picture (Bronfenbrenner and

Crouter, 1982). Briefly, it seems to depend upon both the child's gender and the family's social position—its economic resources. Middle-class and working-class girls with employed mothers do just as well in school as their peers whose mothers are homemakers. Similarly, working-class sons of employed mothers perform just as well in school as their counterparts whose mothers stay home. A number of studies, however, indicate that middle-class boys with mothers who work appear to do less well in school than middle-class boys whose mothers are homemakers. Unfortunately, the studies that have been done do not clearly indicate why this happens. How do the processes vary within these two types of families to produce such results?

Researchers have proposed a variety of reasons why middle-class boys with mothers who work do somewhat less well in school, but there are no definitive answers at present. One notion is that boys may need more supervision than girls, perhaps because they are more likely to fall under the negative influence of a peer group. Working-class boys may be compensated by the fact that their mothers' incomes provide a real improvement in their standard of living—an increase that may not be so appreciable in more affluent families.

Recent research by Bronfenbrenner and his colleagues provides other clues (Bronfenbrenner, Alvarez, and Henderson, 1984). They asked parents of three-year-olds to describe their children in an open-ended interview format. The results are provocative. Mothers who were employed full time and had sons gave the least positive portrayals of their children, and employed mothers of daughters gave the most positive descriptions. In contrast, homemaker mothers were less positive about daughters than they were about sons. What is going on here to produce such a pattern? A key may be the fact that young boys tend to be more active than young girls. For the homemaker, her son's activity level may not bother her. In fact, it may affirm her as a parent. Her son is a healthy child; he's "all boy." For the employed mother, however, the son's activity level may be problematic because she has much more limited time and energy. Over time, she may develop a less positive image of him—and this may mean that she does not provide the attention, encouragement, and support that would ultimately enhance his school achievement. This is purely speculation, of course. But this line of reasoning does point out the potentially important role of the child's temperament.

More research is needed that examines these issues, but we are on the right track when we look for systematic variation in experiences for boys and girls, children in different socioeconomic groups, and so on. For example, there are hints in the research literature that the mother's work schedule makes a difference. Boys whose mothers work part time may not experience any negative consequences of their working.

Not all outcomes of maternal employment are negative. A host of studies point to positive consequences of maternal employment for children. For example, both boys and girls tend to be less sex-stereotyped in their views of men and women if they have mothers in the labor force. In addition, girls benefit in many ways from having an employed mother as a role model. Girls whose mothers work tend to admire their mothers more, have a more positive view of what it means to be female, and are more likely to be independent. Some of these positive characteristics may result from the tendency of employed wives to rely on their daughters for help around the house. In many cases, these girls play an important role in the family economy—and are perceived as making a contribution by other family members.

PATERNAL EMPLOYMENT

Let us now direct our attention to the role of fathers' jobs and their impact on the developing child. Again, early research focused on paternal unemployment. Studies conducted during the Depression, for example, noted that unemployed fathers experienced a decline in authority with their children, especially with their adolescent children. Recently, however, sociologist Glen Elder has had the opportunity to analyze data about children and families that were collected during and after the Depression. He found that teenagers handled the economic disaster fairly well and many benefited from the experience, in part because they were old enough to take an active role in getting the family on its feet, by taking on part-time jobs and so on. Younger children fared less well, especially boys. They were too young to actively help out. In addition, their fathers were frequently irritable, depressed, withdrawn, and frequently inconsistent as disciplinarians. Their sons tended to have social and emotional problems throughout adolescence and young adulthood. Interestingly, these negative effects were much less likely to occur if the husband and wife had a close supportive relationship or if the father and son had established a very close bond before the job loss occurred (see Rockwell and Elder, 1982): a good example of the critical role played by social support during times of stress.

When we look beyond employment status, what does research tell us about the nature of men's work and its effect on children? Traditionally, the husband's occupation has been a primary way researchers have measured a family's social status. Sociologist Melvin Kohn has spent twenty years exploring this issue. When he began, he thought broadly about men's jobs in terms of what they indicated about the family's social position (Kohn, 1969). He found that men hold childrearing values that mirror the qualities linked to success in their lines of work. Blue-collar workers tend to stress obedience and conformity while those in middle-class occupations emphasize independence and initiative.

Other characteristics of fathers' jobs are undoubtedly important. Work absorption, for example, has been linked to fathers being irritable and impatient with their children (Heath, 1976). Work schedules have been identified as a key feature of work. Men on afternoon shifts (3:00–11:00) have difficulty maintaining relationships with their school-aged children because they share so little time together (Mott et al., 1965). In addition, McHale and Huston (in press) found that the number of hours fathers put in on the job is inversely correlated with the extent to which they are involved in leisure and play with their children. A long workday clearly makes a father—or mother—less available as a parent. The father's satisfaction with his job, his workhours, the way in which work affects his mood, and the economic resources provided by the job are all aspects of paternal employment that are finally beginning to be looked at in terms of how they influence children.

Conclusions

It is clear that the work situations of a child's mother and father are an important feature of the child's environment. Children and families depend upon the income parents receive from their work for their economic well-being. Given that families and children need jobs, who should work—mother, father, or both? The answer of course is, "It depends." The key appears to be what combination of roles is preferred by the parents. It is essential that both partners approve of each other's decision, be it to take a job or to remain at home. In the last twenty years, our society has begun to allow women that choice. In the future, if men continue to increase their participation in child care and housework, and as men begin to receive employee benefits such as paternity leave, they too will have options.

It is not enough, however, for husband and wife to reach consensus on who should play what role in the labor force. Their fate depends in part upon the responsiveness of the larger social environment. If a couple decides that both husband and wife will work—an increasingly common choice often made out of necessity—they will need to have support. If they have children, the most important form of support is probably reliable, high-quality, affordable child care. Such care ensures that the child is safe and well cared for when the parents are away at work. This is important not only for infants, toddlers, and preschoolers but for school-aged children as well. We cannot know what effects parental work will have on children unless we know about their daycare arrangements.

If satisfactory care arrangements are found, what else can be done to enhance the relationship between working parents and their families? In her chapter in this volume, Ellen Galinsky describes a number of innovative strategies being implemented in the business world, including flexitime scheduling, employer-sponsored child care, and parenting education in the workplace. There are two additional strategies that emerge directly from the studies summarized in this chapter. The first is that jobs should be made satisfying for the worker/parent. When parents like their jobs, they tend to be happier in their marital relationship and their children appear to function better than when they are not satisfied with their work. Job satisfaction may enhance the individual's self-esteem in a way that makes him or her a better spouse and parent.

A second and related strategy is that jobs should facilitate on individual's adult development. Work can be structured so that it provides workers with new ideas that they can generalize to their own families. For example, Crouter conducted research in a manufacturing plant with a participatory style of management (Crouter, 1984a). Workers were divided into teams that were quite autonomous; they made major decisions and solved problems as a group, rather than being told what to do by a supervisor. During their interviews, these machinists, assembly workers, and managers often mentioned that they had extended the participatory mode of decision making beyond the workplace—to the family. They described coming to the recognition that families are, in a sense, teams and that democratic decision making seemed to work well at home. Given that the child-development literature suggests that children in our culture do benefit from democratic parenting, this is a way in which a feature of work organization might be implemented to enhance children's functioning.

It is ultimately in employers' best interests to have their employees' families functioning smoothly. In the long run, children who misbehave because they are inadequately supervised or marital partners who disapprove of their spouse's work situation are productivity problems. Just as work affects parents and children, parents and children affect the workplace by influencing the employed parents' morale, absenteeism, and productivity (Crouter, 1984b; Voydanoff, 1980). Employees who are worried about family problems represent a problem for employers. Phrased in a more positive way, we all stand to gain when parents are offered solutions that help them to balance work and family roles most effectively.

7 ✳

Family Life and
Corporate Policies

AT A RECENT work and family seminar, the group leader asked the question, "What time do you get up in the morning?"

— "Five A.M."
— "Five-thirty."
— "Six."

"What time do you leave for work?"

— "Six."
— "Six-fifteen."
— "Six-thirty."

"What happens between the time you get up and the time you leave for work?" The forty or so adults in the room began to laugh quietly, with a slight, even bitter embarrassment, the kind of laughter that comes from an experience that was painful at the time but seems funny in retrospect. Then they began to tell their stories.

One father told of a morning when his four-year-old daughter lost her shoes. Amid all the other normal complications of getting two young children dressed, fed, and ready for daycare, he and his wife searched everywhere but the shoes were nowhere to be found. The mother began to go through the house a second time while the father made calls to find someone to take over his carpool to the metal factory where he worked. Because his factory had strict time policies (warnings were issued; after several warnings a worker could be fired), he felt frantic, as did his wife who also had a job tied to the time clock. Eventually they settled for last year's too small shoes, put them on their daughter, and they all rushed out the door. Both parents were late for work, and were censored by their supervisors. When they got home from work, they found a note from their daughter's teacher—it asked them please to buy shoes for their child that fit.

This story illustrates an important facet of today's society: families have changed. The influx of women into the labor force, the dramatic increase in the numbers of working mothers, particularly those with very young children, and the spiraling divorce rate have altered family life in the last two decades (Smith, 1979; Grossman, 1979; Children's Defense Fund, 1982; Axel, 1985). Yet the institutions that families most depend on—the workplace and the schools—have been much slower to change.

In this chapter I will discuss the ways the workplace has begun to respond to the changing family. I have limited its scope to families with children under eighteen who are living at home.

Challenges and Problems of Employed Parents

The following section will detail some of the most important factors that directly or in combination with other factors affect the lives of working parents. Bronfenbrenner and Crouter (1982) and others have noted that these factors have a differential impact on workers depending on several variables. The most important are:

— worksite characteristics: organization, culture, policies
— decision-making characteristics
— community characteristics
— worker/parent characteristics: age, sex, education, job position, marital status
— family characteristics: age of spouse, employment status of spouse, number, age, and sex of children, care of aging parents

For example, the age of the worker's children makes a big difference. Employed workers with young children are more likely to find it difficult to manage both their work and family responsibilities, as do workers who care for aging parents (Galinsky, Roupp, and Blum, 1983; Fernandez, 1985). Other sources note that their children's adolescence can be a stressful time for employed parents, particularly executive fathers (Kiez and Cohen, 1979).

JOB CONDITIONS

Time. Ask any group of working parents to describe their biggest concern and most likely it will be time. Research confirms this: time studies show that when a mother enters the labor force, forty to fifty hours of extra work are added to the family system per week (Hunt and Hunt, 1977). In a census conducted in one plant of a high-technology corporation as part of Bank Street's Corporate Work and Family Life Study, employees were asked to indicate the work condition that most negatively affected their home life. The work condition receiving the highest response (or 25 percent of all respondents) was workhours (Galinsky et al., 1983). Several studies have found that the total hours spent at work each week was the most significant predictor of family strain (Keith and Schafer, 1980; Pleck, Staines, and Lang, 1980; Bohen and Viveros-Long, 1981). Still other studies have determined that the number of workhours in interaction with other factors, such as one's mood at work or lack of job control, is significant (Piotrkowski and Crits-Cristoph, 1982).

The effect of workhours does differ depending on one's sex and on the ages of one's children. Keith and Schafer (1980) found that the number of hours worked was a better predictor of work/ family role strain for men than for women. Likewise, in the University of Michigan's Quality of Employment Survey, excessive workhours were a source of stress for men, whereas, for women, inconvenient workhours were more problematic (Pleck et al., 1980). As one employed mother commented, "How can I discipline and yet maintain a loving relationship with my four-year-old in just three hours a day?" And a father said, "If there could be another ten hours a day, then maybe I could get everything done."

Timing. One of the most problematic aspects of the issue of time is what has been termed schedule incompatibility (Staines and Pleck, 1983). As previously mentioned, Pleck and his colleagues found that schedule conflicts can be particularly troublesome for women.

This stress is intensified if workers are on shift work. The timing of the shift is one important variable. In some cases husbands and wives take shift work so that one is available to care for their children, but then they are rarely able to spend time together (Lein et al., 1974). In other cases a parent may have to leave for work just when the children arrive home from school. Mott, Mann, McLoughlin, and Warwick (1965) found that afternoon shifts resulted in difficulty in parenting while night shifts were associated with marital problems. The negative repercussions of shift work seem to be lessened if workers can select their shifts (De la Mare and Walker, 1968).

The timing of workhours not only affects members of a family and their ability to spend time together; tension is also caused by the clash of an employee's work schedule with events at school. Teacher conferences and school performances usually take place during the workday. Furthermore, school holidays and vacations can create numerous problems for employed parents. Even the hours of the daycare center can be tension-provoking. What happens if a supervisor detains an employee after work for a few minutes or the company institutes compulsory overtime and the daycare center of this employee's child closes promptly at 5:30 P.M.?

Autonomy. Another factor that has emerged as critical is job autonomy. When people feel they have the ability to solve a problem they face and they have commensurate responsibility and decision-making power, they are more likely to be satisfied at work and at home and to have an overall sense of well-being (Piotrkowski and Crits-Cristoph, 1981; Renshaw, 1976; Pearlin and Schooler, 1978). The notion of job control is similar. Workers who have a degree of control over the timing and tasks at work are less subject to stress (Mason and Espinoza, 1983).

Job absorption. Kanter (1977) has pointed to the salience of job absorption in creating family stress. By absorption, she means "occupational pursuits that not only demand the maximum commitment of the worker and define the context for family life; but also implicate other family members and command their direct participation in the work system in either its formal or informal aspects" (p. 26). Several studies have found that when men, particularly those in senior management, are absorbed in their jobs, they are less available for family needs and have poorer relationships with their wives and children (Heath, 1977; Young and Wilmott, 1973). It is important to note that job absorption and job involvement are different. Job involvement refers to the extent to which one's identity is defined by work (Saleh and Hosak, 1976; Lodahl and Kejner, 1965). Both job absorption and job involvement can affect families positively and negatively. On the positive side, they can create the possibility of a role for a nonemployed spouse, such as the executive wife (Kanter, 1977). Piotrkowski (1985) predicts that the greatest difficulties arise for families where individuals are highly involved in and dissatisfied with their jobs.

Relationships at work. The importance of the supervisor relationship has emerged from studies of job stress (House, 1981). In the Bank Street study, employees were asked to select a work condition that had the most negative effect on work. The largest number of respondents selected the supervisor/supervisee relationship (Galinsky et al., 1983). In an open-ended question asking for a workplace change to improve both family life and productivity, a sizeable number of employees wrote about improving the supervisor/supervisee relationship both in terms of their role as a manager, evaluator, and organizer of work tasks and in terms of their sensitivity to the work and family needs of their employees. Fernandez (1985) found a significant relationship between stress at home and work and a boss who was not supportive about the employee's child-care needs.

The relationships with co-workers has also emerged as a significant predictor of stress. In a recent study, Piotrkowski (1985) found that conflict among co-workers, as reported by them, could predict negative mental and physical health outcomes for children up to a year and a half later.

Work location/commuting/relocation. The large majority of employed Americans live and work in different places (Bohen and Viveros-Long, 1981). For those workers who live at a great distance from their workplace or where transportation is not easily arranged or accessible, the length of the workday is extended. Haldi (1977) found that the average time workers spend commuting and working was ten hours more in 1977 than it was in 1940. While some people feel that commuting provides some "time off" or "a time for oneself," others find it exhausting. "I feel like I'm going through a war zone every time I'm on the crowded, overheated train," one parent said. Another reported, "I'm always on edge because I'm so far away from my children. If there were an emergency, it would take me over an hour to get home."

Relocation can cause considerable stress both practically and psychologically to the family, particularly if the spouse works or there are children who have become connected to their community, schools, and friends (Catalyst, 1983; Kamerman, 1983; Renshaw, 1976). Relocation can also cause financial strain. Renshaw (1976) found that choice is a critical factor. If the worker and his or her spouse feel that they themselves have made the decision to move, the aftermath of moving is smoother for all concerned.

FAMILY CONDITIONS

Transitions. Little research attention has been paid to how employed parents make the psychological transition from home to work in the mornings and from work to home in the evenings. Perhaps this is due to the societal myth that work and family constitute separate worlds (Kanter, 1977) and therefore that people are readily able to compartmentalize their two roles. In reality, however, daily transitions are an issue for parents, as Rapoport and Rapoport (1971) determined by interviewing dual-career parents and as Piotrkowski (1979) found when she conducted empirical observations of parents at work and at home. In the work and family seminars conducted by Bank Street for employed parents in corporations, we have seen that parents learn, consciously or not, that the job and the family can require diverse modes of being. There are differences in role, in pacing, in focus, in the amount of feedback one receives, in the way one expresses feelings or acts as an authority. Some parents develop techniques, even ritualistic ways of behaving to help them bridge these differences.

Time for self. Time for self may sound like an ironic topic for employed parents, especially women. Time studies consistently show that working mothers manage by reducing their sleep and eliminating free time (Pleck and Rustad, 1980). Winnett, Neale, and Williams (1982) and Robinson, Converse, and Szalai (1972) found that employed mothers have virtually no free time or time for exercise. At a seminar for working parents at a large corporation, one woman said, "I've had so little time for myself in the past two years that I feel like a tank that's perpetually running on almost empty." Another said, "I'm so needy. If I took some time for myself, I might not be able to stop. I might just get in my car and drive away." Other working mothers note that they must save vacation days not for themselves but for unexpected emergencies—a child becoming ill, a no-show babysitter.

Although free time is also an issue for men, they seem more likely to engage in leisure time or sports activities. Skinner and McCubbin (1982) reported that when men do take time for themselves there is more likely to be an "imbalance" in the family. Perhaps this use of personal time for individual coping further strains the family experiencing overload. Alternatively, this imbalance may arise when husband has the personal time that his wife wants but does not take, resulting in her resentment.

Division of family work. In terms of time spent on various roles, men generally spend more time in work roles while women spend more time in family roles. Taken together, women spend more hours time in both than men (Pleck, 1983). Women do more child care and housework than men, with various studies reporting a range from two to six times as much (Carlson, 1984; Robinson, 1977; Slocum and Nye, 1976; Pleck, 1977, 1983). After close to a decade of researching this issue, Pleck (1983) has found that the proportional (as opposed to the absolute) amount of time that men and women contribute to family work is narrowing because men are doing slightly more housework and child care whereas women are doing less housework. Yogev and Brett (1983) have found that perceptions and expectations are critical factors in this equation. Husbands and wives were more likely to be satisfied with their marriage if they perceive their spouse as doing more than his or her share of child care and housework, even if the actual time spent in such tasks varies from minutes to hours.

Another way to examine family roles is by distinguishing between responsibility for overseeing tasks and the enactment of tasks. In general, women retain the responsibility for overseeing family work (Barnett and Baruch, 1983). This is a complicated issue, one that is linked to the power relationship between the spouses. Russell (1982) found that men are more likely to be substantially involved in the care of their children if the woman has an equal or higher potential for employment and both parents have a philosophical commitment to sharing family responsibilities. Yogman, elsewhere in this volume, has termed women the "gate-keepers" of men's childrearing involvement. As one woman at a work/family seminar stated, "If I gave up being in charge at home, I wouldn't have a comparable amount of responsibility in my job. Society is not at that point yet. So until then, I'll keep my role at home." Women will often say that they want their husbands to help more, though they are often reluctant to ask for the help directly. When the husbands do help, the wives frequently criticize the way their husbands feed the children or clean the house. Perhaps this is a way of minimizing competition between them; but, in the ideal sense, sharing family responsibility means not only sharing the power as well as the work but accepting differences in style.

Dependent care. Child care is one of the main concerns of employed parents. Dana Friedman of the Conference Board tells of a conversation overheard at the beach between two young parents. The mother said to the father, "I'm really enjoying this vacation because I don't have to do the thing I hate the most." "What is it?" he asked, guessing cooking, laundry, housework, commuting, dealing with difficult co-workers. "No," she replied, "it's arranging child care."

This story is revealing because it indicates the complexity of this task both psychologically and practically. Securing child care is not simply a matter of finding one person or program (Morgan, unpublished data). Just figuring out how to find out about the available sources of child care is a job comparable, as one parent said, to learning the rules of a "hidden, somewhat secret society."

Much is unknown about the total child-care picture in the United States because no recent national data have been collected (Ruopp and Travers, 1982; Children's Fund, 1982; Kamerman and Kahn, 1981). It is known, however, that the supply of quality and affordable care in no way meets the demand, especially in the areas of infant/toddler care and after-school care (Blank, 1984; Seligson, Genser, Gannet, and Gray, 1983). It is also known that child care forms a two-tiered system: care paid for by middle-income parents and subsidized care for low-income parents. Recent federal, state, and local budget cuts have drastically reduced the supply of care for the children of the working poor, who are more likely to be left to care for themselves or to have been moved to substandard daycare arrangements (Blank, 1984; Children's Fund, 1984).

Once parents do find child care, it is often not simply one provider. Kamerman (1980) has documented the fact that employed parents develop an intricate "package" of different types of care for each child for different times of the day. For many, this package carries a high price (Ruopp and Travers, 1982); for others, these arrangements are tenuous.

One of the most frequently asked policy questions is, What is the impact of various kinds of child-care arrangements on productivity? No such studies on productivity per se have been conducted to date, but there are several notable large-scale studies that investigate stress, absenteeism, and unproductive worktime for men and for women with different-aged children. In a study of 8,121 employees in 33 companies and agencies in Portland, Oregon, Emlen and Koren (1984) found that men whose children remained at home with their spouse had an absenteeism rate that was comparable to employees with no children; women whose children were cared for outside the home or in self- or sibling care had the highest absenteeism rates. "This range was 65 percent higher in days missed—278 percent higher in leaving work earlier and 210 percent higher in interruptions" (p. 6). Emlen and Koren also found that stress (as experienced during the prior four weeks) was significantly related to how families arranged their child care. For example, half of the women who relied on their children to care for themselves or 46 percent of those who used out-of-home care experienced stress. Among employed parents with children under twelve, 47 percent of the women and 28 percent of the men reported some child-care stress. These figures did not differ for families with younger children or for those with higher incomes. The researchers state, "These proportions of the work force reporting stress are all the more significant when it is recognized how brief a slice of life is represented by a 4-week period in which the stress could occur" (p. 7).

Fernandez (1985), in a study of 5,000 workers in 5 corporations, investigated stress, unproductive worktime, and absenteeism, and found that the age of children was most significant. In addition, he found that caring for a sick child was the cause of absenteeism by 56 percent of the women who were absent from one to three times during the previous year, by 78 percent of those with four to six days missed, and by an astounding 82 percent of those absent more than six days.

There has been less research on how work conditions affect the care of aging parents (Pirie, 1985). It is known, however, that women by and large provide this care and that, because of their entrance into the labor force, the declining birth rate, and the increase in the number of aging people, it is projected that fewer family members will be available to provide care for the aging.

WORK/FAMILY INTERFERENCE

A structural interference. The degree to which work and family life interfere or conflict with each other has been termed work/family interference (Pleck, 1979). In the University of Michigan Quality of Employment Survey, a third of the nationally representative respondents reported moderate to severe conflict between work and family life (Pleck et al., 1978).

This first interference can be of two kinds. The first is structural interference, or the actual time constraints imposed by the demands of both roles (Hughes, 1985). Most of the research on structural interference has investigated job-to-family interference focusing on time constraints.

Virtually no research has been done on how employees manage children or other family concerns from the workplace, yet this issue is important to both employees and employers. Workers often have to deal with emergencies, large and small, while at work: they have to arrange a different carpool ride for a child, make a doctor's appointment for an elderly parent, or deal with a family conflict, such as a teenager who is suspected of drinking or using drugs. For those employees who have children who care for themselves after school, there can be a period of tension until the child telephones to say he or she is safe at home (this applies to employees who have access to a telephone—many don't). Employers know this as the "3:15 syndrome,"—sometimes noting that "productivity slumps at this time."

Work/family interference has been found to have negative consequences. Pleck (1979) found a negative correlation between the perception of work/family interference and job satisfaction, overall well-being, and family adjustment. Furthermore, he found that women are more vulnerable to work/family conflict than men (Pleck, unpublished).

Psychological interference. Piotrkowski (1979) documented that affective states spill over from work to family and from family to work. Spillover refers to both mood and to energy level (Hughes, 1985). Crouter (1984) has found that negative feelings at the end of the workday are associated with more irritability at home. A recent longitudinal study by Belsky, Perry-Jenkins, and Crouter (1985) found that during the transition to parenthood, those husbands and wives who experienced high levels of negative work/family spillover reported an increase in marital conflict.

A related concept is role overload. Rapoport and Rapoport (1971) have noted that employed parents can experience role overload, the feeling that there is too much to do and not enough time or energy. Others have termed this state "energy deficit" (Piotrkowski, 1979) or "role strain" (Bohen and Viveros-Long, 1981).

STRESS BUFFERS

There are a number of variables, identified in previous studies, that can act as buffers between work and family conditions and positive or negative outcomes. One such variable is socioeconomic status. The money to purchase services has been found significant in reducing the conflict between the demands at home and at work (Belle, 1982). Other stress buffers are social support, coping style, and expectations.

Social support. Social support means informal help from one's spouse, children, relatives, neighbors, or friends as well as more formal help from community agencies, religious organizations, or counselors. Social support has been consistently found to lessen the effects of work/family stress and to contribute to health and well-being (Cobb, 1979; Unger and Powell, 1980; Gottlieb, 1978; Belle, 1982; Pearlin and Schooler, 1978).

Coping style. Coping has been described as the adaptational techniques used by an individual to master a major psychological threat and its attendant negative feelings. Lazarus and Launier (1978) have proposed two classes of coping strategies: problem-focused, or direct action aimed at eliminatory or changing the anticipated harm; and emotion-focused, a cognitive maneuver aimed at lessening the stress by reinterpreting it. In addition to identifying specific coping strategies, an individual's general pattern of coping can be described as active or passive. Lazarus and Launier state that "the ways people cope with stress [may be] even more important to overall morale, social functioning and health/illness than the frequency and severity of episodes of stress themselves" (p. 308). In their research on coping with job stress, Shinn et al. (in press) found that group strategies related more significantly to positive individual coping efforts. They also found that problem-focused coping was more effective.

Expectations. In all the issues that employed parents face, expectations—images, conscious or not, of the way things are supposed to go or people are supposed to behave—are a powerful factor. Mason and Espinoza (1983) have found that family stress is more likely if family members have different expectations, particularly in relation to whether the mother should be employed. Research on the impact of a mother's work on children has singled out the mother's belief that she should be employed as a critical variable in relation to positive outcomes for children (Yarrow et al., 1962; Hock, 1979; Belsky, Steinberg, and Walker, 1982; Hoffman, 1982). How the reality and timing of one's work life fits one's expectations or hopes is also significant in overall satisfaction (Piotrokowski, 1979; Levinson et al., 1978).

Expectations are shaped by the indiviual's life experience and by cultural norms. In Bank Street's work with parents in corporate seminars, four parental images repeatedly emerge: supermother, superfather, superbaby, and quality time. The superperson has it all, does it all. The supermother is able to work a forty-hour week, keep the house clean and neat, entertain, keep physically fit by jogging or taking aerobics, and have a meaningful relationship with the superfather, who is both productive and nurturing and who fully shares in the work of running the household. The superbaby—brilliant, all-American, and normal—happily waves goodbye to his or her parents while going off to a toddler gym. Of course, the superparents have problem-free time with their children, the essence of quality time.

Parents feel the strain of unmet expectations when their house is disorganized and hectic, and when their quality time turns into a referee match between tired and squabbling children. One parent said that, if her children raised their voices in the evening, her palms would get all sweaty as she would think, "There goes my quality time for tonight."

Family-Responsive Corporate Policies

There are a number of innovative family-responsive corporate programs that address the problems that employed parents face. Before I describe them I would like to suggest a word of caution. First, there can be a great deal of variety in the way a program is implemented, depending largely on the sensibilities of the specific manager. Second, family-responsive programs have been instituted in different corporations for a variety of complex reasons, and the motivation that such a program would be "good for families" rarely predominates. Corporations develop programs that are first and foremost "good for the corporation" at the least cost— that is, those seen as increasing productivity, improving recruitment and retention, and reducing absenteeism. Bohen (1983) summarizes an Aspen Institute seminar on family-related corporate policy attended by executives by saying that "there have to be bottom-line reasons for corporations to change what they do" (p. 34).

While numerous Americans admire the governmental family policies in European countries, such as lengthy maternity/paternity leaves and cash payments to subsidize the cost of raising children, it should be understood that these policies were generally not instituted for pro-family reasons. Their impetus was frequently to raise the birth rates or to attract women into the labor market or to keep them out (Bohen, 1983; Kamerman and Kahn, 1981). The argument, however, that the American government does not have such policies because we believe that government should not interfere with family life does not withstand scrutiny. We have frequently instituted governmental programs and policies for low-income families as well as policies related to the education of children.

In contrast to the European countries where government programs predominate in the social welfare system, the United States places a much greater stress on what Kamerman and Kingston (1982) term a "corporate social welfare system." This system, however, is not comprehensive; it serves one segment of the population, those who work for large employers.

If one defines a small business as the Small Business Association does—a business employing fewer than five hundred employees—99 percent of all businesses fall into this category. Almost half the workers in the United States work for companies that employ fewer than one hundred people. These people do not generally receive the benefits and services that large corporations provide or that sometimes have been won by union initiative (Kamerman, 1983). Factors that have led to the development of corporate family programs include the following: large size of company, young entrepreneurial leadership, products or services related to family, a high percentage of women employees, and a prime mover within the corporation who is committed to bringing about change (Friedman, 1983).

As I describe family-responsive programs, a term coined by Kamerman (1983), it will be clear that the same corporations are being mentioned again and again. As Friedman (1984) states, a select number of corporations have developed a large number of innovative programs.

MECHANISMS FOR INSTITUTING FAMILY-RESPONSIVE POLICY

Corporate programs and policies are generally instigated by top management, often in response to an internal problem that is of concern (Levinson, Spohn, and Molinari, 1972) or by hearing about an initiative at another company that will prevent an anticipated problem (Friedman, 1983). It is far less frequent for a work/family program to be initiated by nonmanagerial workers. A number of corporations have set up orderly feedback mechanisms to learn more about their employees' needs.

Need assessment. Need assessments are surveys that gather information on the employee population.

Task force. A task force is a group, usually consisting of management and workers, that is formed to consider a specific issue and design a solution.

Quality circles. Quality circles are on-going, permanent groups of employees, typically representing diverse job levels, who form work teams that meet to discuss and resolve work-related problems (Ouchi, 1981; Solman and Friedman, 1982; Simon and Mares, 1982).

Face-to-face groups. In these sessions, the top-level supervisor meets with all the staff and answers questions that are submitted in person or in writing.

Suggestion box. Regular columns in the company newspaper can also serve as a vehicle for employees to initiate questions on diverse topics, including the company's plans for dealing with employees' work and family problems.

Electronic mail. Several companies are thinking about using their computer capacity to meet work/family needs. For example, an employee needing a tutor for a grade-school child might use an electronic mail system to see if there are other employees able to take on this job. Electronic mail can supplement question and answer columns to provide information on company programs and policies.

CORPORATE POLICIES RELATED TO WORKHOURS

Flexitime. Flexitime stands for flexible work hours: employees choose their own arrival and departure times within the limits determined by the company. Nollen (1982) notes that schedules vary along three dimensions: daily versus periodic setting of the work schedule; variable versus constant length of workday (whether employees can credit time from one day to the next); and core time, the hours, usually during the middle of the workday, when all employees are required to be present.

In 1980, 11.9 percent of all nonfarm workers, or 7.6 million people, were on flexitime (Nollen, 1982). While the impact of flexitime has generally been positive for the worker and corporation (Nollen, 1982; Kirk, 1981), Bohen and Viveros-Long (1981) found it was less successful for working parents. They report, "The primary group whose family lives were expected to benefit from more flexible work schedules, namely employed mothers, did not report less stress than mothers on standard schedule" (p. 120). Because of the nature of this study (it was done as a survey), the in-depth reasons behind this finding were not clear. The authors do suggest that the modest time changes in this flexitime program may simply not have been enough to help working mothers. Other flexitime studies report contradictory findings: there is more available family time and more ease in making child-care arrangements (Winnett and Neal, 1981).

Compressed workweek. A compressed workweek is a full-time job that is scheduled in less than five days a week. The schedules more frequently used are four 10-hour days; three 12-hour days; four-and-a-half-day workweek with four 9-hour days and one 4-hour day; and the 5/4-9 plan with alternating five-day weeks and four-day weeks with 9 hours a day (Nollen, 1982). In 1980, 2.7 percent of all full-time nonfarm workers, or 1.7 million people, were on compressed workweeks (Nollen, 1982). The use of the compressed workweek has been shown to have both a positive and negative outcome for the worker and for the corporation. Workers can have more time to be with their families but can be more tired after working the long days (Nollen, 1982; Staines and Pleck, 1983).

Part-time work. Part-time work is defined as a job of less than thirty-five hours a week. Permanent, professional part-time work has job security, advancement possibilities, and benefit coverage. In 1982, according to Plewes (1984), one in five of all workers, or 18 million people, worked under thirty-five hours a week and the majority, or 70 percent, did so by choice. Seventy percent of all voluntary part-time workers are women. Few part-timers have professional status or receive prorated benefits. Unions have traditionally been opposed to part-time work because it has been seen as a way of undermining the union's bargaining strength.

Part-time work is frequently seen as a solution to work/family problems by parents. In the General Mills Survey by Harris and his associates (1981), 42 percent of the respondents felt that part-time work with full-time benefits would help "a great deal" in reducing work/family tensions.

After completing three surveys, the New York State Council on Children and Families (1983) has developed a program to increase the use of part-time work for state employees. Most notable is their concept of what has been termed V-Time or voluntary reduced worktime. Under such a plan, an employee can reduce his or her time for a limited period while retaining seniority status and benefits. The concept of V-Time was originally developed in 1976 by the Service Employees International Union in Santa Clara, California.

Job sharing. Job sharing means that two people share one position: the workers are part-time, the position full-time. Job sharing has been seen as a way to help parents manage work and family life more efficiently (Olmsted and Smith, 1983; Meier, 1979). Reports indicate that the most widespread use is for teachers and clericals, but there is some indication that its use is spreading to groups where it was thought unworkable in the past, such as managers and lawyers (Collins, 1984).

Improvement of shift work. Shift work can be fixed (that is, always at the same time) or rotating. The worker under a rotating schedule moves from a day to an afternoon to a night shift on a regular basis. In the Bank Street research, a number of workers noted that the timing of shift work caused problems in fulfilling family responsibilities—especially when they were scheduled for the afternoon shift and had to leave just as their children arrived home from school (Galinsky et al., 1983). On the other hand, shift work is frequently used by two-parent working families as a way for both parents to share in childrearing without having to rely on outside care (Lein et al., 1974). The major improvement in shift work for families would be to provide workers with a choice, so that they could determine their own schedules.

Improvement of overtime policies. The issue of overtime is complex. While workers may want more overtime because it increases their income, they may object to being forced to work overtime. Problems can occur for families when overtime is on an emergency or last-minute basis, and when workers are penalized if they refuse to stay. Another problem is mandatory overtime: for example, a system where employees must work twelve hour days or on Saturdays/Sundays. Making overtime voluntary, preferably with advance notice, would improve its use for families.

Personal days. The purpose of personal days is to extend the definition of sick days (a specified amount of paid leave for sickness) to days off that can be used for personal or family reasons. This means that the employee can use this paid leave to take care of a sick child, an aging parent, or tend to other personal or family problems. At present only a third to a half of workers are covered with paid sick leaves (Kamerman, 1983). A Catalyst study (1981) of 374 of the Fortune 1300 companies indicated that 28 percent of the companies surveyed did provide personal days. At corporate work and family seminars, employed parents admit that if their employer does not permit personal days, they are forced to lie, saying they are ill in order to remain at home with a sick child.

Time bank. Under this program, each employee has a certain number of available paid hours to spend away from work during the year. The employee can take time off in two- to three-hour increments. A time bank offers employed parents the flexibility to attend teacher conferences or other functions at their children's schools, or to take care of other personal responsibilities. At Becton Dickinson's plant at Orangeburg, New York, the Oil, Chemical and Atomic Worker's Union was successful in negotiating a time bank.

CORPORATE POLICIES RELATED TO WORKPLACE

Flexiplace. Toffler (1980) has proposed an image of the future in which there is a shift away from the centralized corporate workplace to a more decentralized cottage industry, with increasing numbers of people working in their homes and neighborhoods. While certain professionals and executives have always had the opportunity to work at home, and this flexibility has been enhanced by advances in technology that connect people no matter where they are physically based, the use of flexiplace or working at home is not widely used. Continental Illinois Bank in Chicago has experimented with placing word processors in employees' homes (Axel, 1985).

Flexiplace has numerous advantages: eliminating commuting time and providing flexibility for the worker to take care of family needs. There are also disadvantages: workers have reported feeling isolated; some workers are paid in a piecework manner, often without benefits; and although the vision of working at home while caring for children may sound appealing, the reality of a child's needing attention while the parent has work to do can be frustrating.

Relocation assistance. A number of companies have found that it is to their benefit to think about the personal and family needs of employees who are being transferred. This is done either by the in-house personnel division or by a subcontract with a consulting firm.

The major form of service provided by corporations is economic. Most large corporations now pay the costs associated with moving: trips to look for housing, temporary living expenses, storage, direct moving costs, and sometimes the purchase of furniture and appliances. Some corporations also help employees by buying and then reselling their old home or developing policies to help in the purchase of a new home (Kamerman, 1983). Chase Manhattan Bank has a relocation allowance for expatriates that consists of a proportion of the employee's salary to be used at the employee's discretion. Their expatriate policy also includes pay for vacations, trips for family members to visit the employee at the new location, and language lessons.

Several companies have created programs to help the spouse of the relocated worker. Merck and Company was instrumental in developing a consortium of corporations that form a network for job assistance and placement for the spouse. This service is important because, as Runzheimer (1979) found, one fifth of the executives who refused to relocate made this decision because of their employed spouse. For other companies, assistance is in the form of counseling for the spouse. Baxter Travenol Laboratories and Burger King also plan for the needs of children. They have developed care packages for children that include such things as scrapbooks, address books, and stationery.

BENEFIT PROGRAMS

Flexible benefits. It is important to put innovative programs within the context of the general benefit picture. Not all workers are covered with what is considered a standard benefit package. Kamerman (1983) has done an excellent job in assembling information about coverage as it currently exists. The Bureau of Labor Statistics (1984) reports that 97 percent of all workers have individual health insurance, with close to three quarters of that coverage paid for by the employer. The Bureau of the Census (1983) showed, however, that less than half of American households have the more costly family health coverage paid for by the employer.

Similarly, the Bureau of Labor Statistics (1982) reveals that 84 percent of the firms surveyed have retirement pension plans; other studies, summarized by Kamerman (1983), put those figures in the 40-50 percent range. Kamerman makes the important point that not much is known about benefit coverage provided by small businesses.

Flexible benefits became possible in 1970 under section 125 of the Internal Revenue Code, though most have been instituted since 1982 (Friedman, 1985). They are seen as a large step forward in corporate programs. Whereas the typical benefit plan is designed as if there were only one employed adult in the household, under a flexible plan an employee can develop an individual package that fits his or her particular needs and eliminates duplication. For example, if two parents are working, both do not need health insurance coverage. One of the parents can trade off this benefit for such things as cash compensation, dental care, dependent care, or life insurance.

Companies with flexible benefit plans differ on the ranges of choices offered: some have core coverage (generally consisting of health insurance, disability life insurance, retirement pension, and vacation) with options. In other companies, an employee can tailor a more individual plan.

The overall response to flexible benefit plans has been positive. In an American Can survey about their flexible program, reported in Kamerman (1983), 90 percent of the employees liked to choose new benefits on a yearly basis and 75 percent judged the program as "very good" to "excellent." American Can's plan, however, required a great deal of administrative time to set up and company-wide education to use it. There are more than 150 employers with flexible benefit programs (Friedman, 1985). They include TRW, Pepsico, and Proctor and Gamble.

Flexible benefits are, however, controversial in the unionized sector. There is the concern that the older or weaker workers will not be served as well. For example, if younger workers do not select retirement benefits, the pension fund may erode. Furthermore, a current governmental debate is brewing about flexible benefits: Should benefits, now tax-free, be taxed?

Salary-reduction plans and flexible spending accounts. Salary-reduction plans became possible after new tax legislation in 1978. Under such plans, employees can reduce a certain percentage of their income and place pretax dollars in flexible spending accounts (FSA) to be used to reimburse certain predetermined expenses not included in the regular benefit package, such as dental bills or child care. These plans can exist as part of a flexible benefit program in which the employer contributes benefit dollars or can exist separately, that is, as a stand-alone salary-reduction plan.

Because the IRS has taken a long time to define the boundaries of usage, these plans had a slow start-up. Furthermore a recent ruling by the IRS has been seen as a temporary setback for the more open ended flexible spending accounts. It was decided that the money in salary reduction accounts must be used up by the year's end or be forfeited. The Conference Board has recently found that the salary reduction plans are becoming widely used with as many as 800 FSAs in operation.

Dependent care assistance plans. Section 129 of the IRS code of Economic Recovery Tax Act of 1981 allows employers to pay for child care with tax-deductible dollars by reimbursing the employee or by paying the care provider directly. Approximately 150 companies have currently established DCAP programs (Money, 1985).

Another provision in this legislation has been important to working parents: the child-care tax credit. This credit is calculated on a sliding scale based on income and number of children. Those earning under $10,000 before taxes are eligible for a credit of 30 percent of their costs, with a maximum credit of $720 for one child or dependent and $1440 for two or more. For those who earn over $28,000 or more, 20 percent of their costs can be claimed with a maximum credit of $480 for one child and $960 for two or more.

Reimbursement programs. Under reimbursement programs, the company reimburses the employee for a portion or the full cost of child care. These programs are either part of a benefit plan or exist as an additional service. In some cases, the parent presents the company with a bill or a canceled check and is reimbursed. In other cases a voucher is the medium of exchange. The employee is given a voucher by the employer which he or she gives to the care provider, who in turn is paid by the employer. The National Employer Supported Child Care Project (Burud, Aschbacher, and McCroskey, 1984) identified seventeen companies that have reimbursement programs. A recent study by Friedman (1985) found little change—fewer than twenty-five companies have voucher programs.

The advantage of reimbursement or voucher programs is that the choice of child care remains in the parents' hands; the company stays out of the daycare business. The expense of these programs depends on the amount of subsidy offered. These programs help parents afford child care, which is estimated to be one of the highest costs a family must bear after food and housing (Ruopp and Travers, 1982). Examples of companies providing reimbursement programs are the Polaroid Corporation and the Ford Foundation. Austin Families has developed a voucher program for its city's school bus drivers.

Improved vacation policies. The standard vacation for American workers is two weeks. According to Kamerman (1983), three fourths of employees with less than a year of service receive only a week off. Only after ten years is the worker's vacation time increased to three weeks, though some companies provide three weeks for those employees with a tenure of five to seven years. One improvement in vacation policies would be the lengthening of vacations. Another critical improvement would be to allow employees the opportunity to schedule the timing of their vacations so that they could plan for family needs, such as making sure their vacation coincides with the vacations of other family members.

Improved leaves. In the United States, maternity leaves are provided through the disability benefits of employers or through the disability benefits that have been mandated in five states (Kamerman, Kahn, and Kingston, 1983). The Pregnancy Discrimination Act of 1978 has determined that pregnancy must be treated like any other worker disability; that is, if a corporation provides disability benefits, pregnant women must be included. Furthermore, this act eliminated the restrictions on when a woman must leave work before child bearing and specified that the woman's job must be protected, although companies differ in their interpretation of "the same or comparable job."

Kamerman, Kahn, and Kingston (1983) have found that the standard American coverage is six to eight weeks, with some companies allowing as little as four weeks. One powerful finding of their recent study is their estimate that only 40 percent of all working women are covered with maternity-leave benefits. Because so many women work for companies that do not provide disability coverage, American policy is strikingly different from virtually every other industrialized country in which maternity leaves are mandated by law (Kamerman, 1983; Hewlitt, 1983). The net effect of the 1978 law has been both positive and negative. One negative repercussion is that some companies have eliminated unpaid leaves for everyone because, as they say, they do not want to offer it to men.

It is clear that the best way to improve maternity leave is to lengthen it, combining paid with unpaid leave for six months, a year, or a year and a half, including job security and no loss of seniority. While some companies are concerned that such leaves would be costly in terms of staff coverage and might create an internal lobby for men to have paternity leaves (Kamerman et al., 1983), several companies such as Merck have developed longer maternity leaves without undue reported difficulty. Silverman (1984) has speculated that better maternity policies would not only "bond" the employee to the company, thereby increasing loyalty, but would certainly provide a healthier beginning for mother and child—ultimately, a preventive measure. A very promising new direction is a transitional period of part-time work after maternity leave, easing back to full-time work. A few organizations such as the Port Authority in New York and New Jersey are considering this.

Although paternity leaves have received a great deal of media attention, there are few in existence. Pleck (unpublished) argues for a redefinition of leave, noting that most fathers take time off around the birth of a child through an informal understanding with the supervisor or through sick, vacation, or unpaid leave days. Among the organizations offering more extended paternity leaves are Bank Street College and CBS.

An equally small number of companies provide adoption leave or coverage of costs (Kamerman, 1983). Several adoptive parenting groups have begun to campaign for this benefit, and their use may begin to spread.

Preventive health benefits. Preventive health care is becoming widely seen as an important means to cut high insurance costs for companies. Numerous corporations have on-site doctors and nurses for regular medical care or job emergencies. Employers pay for memberships (generally for executives) at health clubs. *House and Garden* magazine is one company that has recently instituted this benefit. In other companies, cardiovascular fitness programs are being developed. Johnson and Johnson offers a stop-smoking program, and a number of companies have built jogging tracks. Pepsico has jogging tracks, Nautilus equipment, and gyms that include such classes as aerobics.

FAMILY-RESPONSIVE SERVICES

Employee assistance. Employee Assistance Programs (EAP) or counseling services were begun in the last several decades to provide assistance to alcoholic employees. Their use has spread to include any number of issues that may affect a worker's job performance: marital discord, care of aging parents, child-care difficulties, other work or family problems. It is estimated that there are currently five thousand such programs in the country (Leavitt, 1983). Some companies have in-house services. Citibank, for example, has a comprehensive staff advisory service that provides information, including child care or legal assistance, referral, short-term counseling, and group workshops, at no cost to the employee. Other companies such as Phillip Morris bring outside consultants on site.

Leavitt (1983) indicates that although few systematic evaluations have been conducted, employers believe that EAP programs are cost-effective. On the whole, employees feel that these services are extremely helpful, though some companies report that they are not serving all those who might need the service. This occurs for a variety of reasons, including the difficulty that some employees have in asking for help, a fear of bureaucracy, or distrust of going to the company with personal problems.

CHILD-CARE SUPPORT

The number of corporate initiatives related to child care is increasing. Burud and colleagues (1984) noted a growth rate of 395 percent between 1978 and 1982. In 1978, 105 company day-care centers were identified; in 1982 the range of services being provided had increased and included 415 companies. The Conference Board estimates that in 1985 over 1200 companies were involved.

Resource and referral. The fastest growing corporate child-care initiative is resource and referral (R&R) with, according to Conference Board estimates, 500 companies offering this service in 1985. R&R (as opposed to information and referral) has two distinct components: the provision of counseling services to help parents use information in order to make child-care choices; and the provision of money or resources to increase the quantity or improve the quality of the daycare supply.

An employee calls or visits an R&R service to locate child care. Typically, the employee is interviewed about the kind, location, and cost of care desired. The R&R staff member then provides the employee with a list of several options that fit the employee's criteria. In general, R&R services include only programs or providers that are legally licensed or registered. It is customary for R&R services never to recommend one program over another. There is an allegiance, legal and ethical, to having the parent make the decision. R&R services do give parents guidelines for making choices and then have follow-up procedures to determine what selection employees have made and how satisfied they are with their choice.

Employers have different methods of providing R&R. Some contract out to local agencies. In New York City, for example, Child Care Inc. has contracts with numerous corporations including Time, International Paper, Bristol-Myers, and the Port Authority. Several companies have developed an in-house R&R capacity, as Citibank has done, or have hired consultants on site. The latter method has been used by Steelcase in Grand Rapids, Michigan. Two local daycare specialists not only provide R&R but in the process have increased the quantity and quality of family daycare in the area. They have a lending library and a newsletter and provide training to care providers.

In the summer of 1984, IBM announced R&R to its 220,000 employees in the United States. They have retained Work/Family Directions, a joint venture of Wheelock College and Rodgers & Associates, to coordinate a national network of R&R agencies and to increase the quantity of child care in all of their sites throughout the country. They have been quite successful in expanding the supply of child care as well as building a national network of R&R services.

BankAmerica has also intitiated an important advance in this field by beginning and becoming the first funder of the California Child Care Initiative. Its purposes are to:

— conduct a market survey to assess local supply and demand and identify the types of care most needed
— recruit and screen potential new daycare providers
— work with existing workers who could expand or adjust their capacity to meet demand better
— train new and existing providers in delivery of good care as well as effective business management
— link providers to sources of financing

— provide technical assistance to new providers in meeting state licensing requirements and local codes (Mans, 1984)

Companies find that R&R is a low-cost commitment. Although some companies report that the start-up is slow or the use is lower than predicted (between 2 to 3 percent of all employees on site on the average), employers are generally quite pleased about the decision to provide this service. Family advocates, however, sometimes maintain that companies select R&R as a way of avoiding a greater involvement in the child-care issue, while others say that it is a first step in corporate involvement and may lead to other programs and policies. There are some companies that are thinking of expanding R&R to include resource and referral about other family needs, such as the care of aging parents or relatives.

Support for community care. Another form of company aid to child care is the provision of support to existing local programs. In some cases, companies give money to a center; in return, a certain number of slots are held for employees or employees are given preferential admission. Another form of subsidy is corporate payment for a number of slots within a program for employees' children. This differs from reimbursement because the financial transaction is between the company and the provider; with reimbursement, the parent pays and is refunded.

Consortiums. Another corporate initiative is a consortium of companies that band together to create a center. Examples include the Broadcasters Child Development Center in Washington D.C., developed by seven radio and television stations; the Children's Village in Philadelphia, developed by garment workers; and the Prospect Hill Parents' and Children's Center for a group of companies off Route 128 in Waltham, Massachusetts. Another example is the infant/toddler program developed by Hackensack Medical Center and the *Bergen Record* in New Jersey.

Provision of start-up costs. When Merck and Company, in Rahway, New Jersey, was approached by a number of employees in need of child care, they developed a unique solution. Deciding that the company did not want to run a center itself, money was given to parent employees to develop their own program, the Employees' Center for Young Children. This approach is not problem-free.

Without ongoing corporate support, the care is expensive and therefore primarily serves higher-paid employees. The center has a waiting list of over sixty families. The solution is, however, a way for a corporation to help while not being directly involved.

On-site care. When corporate initiatives for child care are discussed, most people think of on-site child care. In fact, as this chapter indicates, there is a wide spectrum of child-care supports a company can offer. Out of eighteen proposed benefits in the Quality of Employment Survey of 1977, on-site child care was least selected by respondents (Quinn and Staines, 1979); but in the large study by Fernandez (1985), workers voiced a preference for on- or near-site child care. The Conference Board estimates that there were 150 on- or near-site corporate centers, 400 centers in hospitals for employees' children, and 30 public agency centers in 1985.

There are several reasons why parents do not desire on-site child care: some parents want to have neighborhood care; they are not eager to travel with young children; they fear becoming overly committed to the company (Galinsky and Hooks, 1977). The disincentives for companies include concern about liability and the equity issue, that is, the high cost of serving a relatively small number of employees. Because daycare is labor-intensive (even though daycare workers are generally underpaid), quality care is expensive (Ruopp and Travers, 1982).

On the positive side, on-site child care reduces the separation between work and family life. The child can know about the parent's work, the parent can be a part of the child's day; mothers can nurse, and parents and children can have lunch together (Galinsky and Hooks, 1977). It is important for employers to realize that on-site care is only one of numerous options and must fit the needs and desires of the employee population for it to work.

There has been some research about the advantages of on-site child care for employees. Most of these surveys have been based on manager perception. Perry (1978) found that most managers believe their programs are effective in accomplishing such goals as attracting new employees, lowering absenteeism, and improving attitudes toward the employer. Burud and her colleagues (1984) found the highest perceived effects of employer-supported child care to be the ability to improve employee morale, attract talented employees, and serve as good public relations. Magid (1983) also found the greatest perceived benefits to be recruitment and employee morale.

Intermedics studied the impact of its center in Freeport, Texas, and found a reduction in turnover, with a gain of 3700 workhours (Friedman, 1983). The Northside Child Development Center in Minneapolis also conducted a twenty-month study of a sample of mothers matched to two control groups and found significantly lower absentee and turnover rates for the daycare mothers (Milkovich and Gomez, 1976). In the later study, however, the researchers did not investigate the kind of child care the control groups used or previous levels of absenteeism (Miller, 1984). Some of the older and better known on-site centers include Zale Corporation, Stride Rite Shoe Company, Corning Glass, Abt Associates, and Hoffmann-La Roche.

Sick-child and travel care. Finding care for sick children is one of the most difficult problems that employed parents face. Some companies, as already noted, provide personal days so that parent and child can be together. This is deemed the most comfortable solution for both when the child is very ill. A few companies are exploring the development of sick-child facilities, although problems of contagion, cost, and providing unfamiliar care to a sick child are often inhibiting. The Berkeley Sick Child Program in California provides a trained worker to come into the home. Parents pay for this service on a sliding scale from no fee to $3.50 an hour (Burud et al., 1984).

One of the most exciting sick-child programs is being piloted by 3M in St. Paul, Minnesota. With funds from the Contribution Board, the company has made arrangements for sick care with health workers through a local concern, Home Health Plus. Moreover, the company contributes to the cost of the care on a sliding scale based on family income. The cost of the care is $8 an hour; the parent pays from $2 to $4 per hour per child.

Employees also face child-care problems when they travel for their jobs. This problem has recently come to the attention of Hewlett Packard, which has a task force investigating the issue, particularly for its single working-mother employees.

In-kind donations. In-kind donations are not usually included when corporate programs are discussed, although they provide an important contribution to child care. In Austin, Texas, an Adopt-A-School program has been developed in which employees regularly volunteer time during the workday to tutor children. Other corporations lend staff members to help child-care organizations. The Orange and Rockland Utility in New York has donated the expertise of its public relations staff to the Rockland Council for Young Children and has printed brochures for the council. Other in-kind corporate donations to child care include materials (say scrap paper) or products (cameras).

Corporate initiatives. The senior managers of many companies have been instrumental in initiating daycare programs, particularly for after-school care. For example, in Houston, Texas, a number of executives have been working with public schools to begin after-school programs in all sixty elementary schools. The resulting program, now in fifteen schools, is administered by United Way with parents paying on a sliding scale.

TRAINING PROGRAMS

Work and family seminars. In a recent review by Catalyst (1984), it is estimated that the number of workplaces offering work and family seminars is growing: approximately one thousand corporations offer this service. While varying in location, format, length, and content, these seminars share a common purpose: "to address the work and family concerns of employees." They are unique in being able to address issues for all employees, from single workers to those with aging parents.

Seminars take place at lunchtime, after work, or for a full or half day. The topics addressed include time management, the impact of working on children, finding and evaluating child care, managing children from the workplace, and family communication. Seminars offer employers a way to find out about and serve employees' needs in a preventive manner at a proportionally minimal cost. Company officials believe they increase job performance. For the employee, they offer the solace of knowing they are not alone in facing work/family problems as well as the opportunity to develop practical solutions and support.

Some of the companies that provide seminars include Exxon, Citibank, Phillip Morris, *Time*, Home Box Office, Bristol-Myers, Hoffmann-La Roche, Pfizer, and International Paper. Seminars are provided by freelance consultants or by educational organizations such as Wheelock College and Bank Street College.

Seminars for families. Local 8-149 of the Oil, Chemical and Atomic

Workers has created a slightly new version of the working-parent seminars. They hold a seminar on a Saturday at a country retreat. The union member, spouse, and children all participate in recreation, sports, and educational programs. For example, the school-age children and their parents discuss practical strategies for coping when children care for themselves and younger siblings after school. Phoenix Mutual in Hartford, Connecticut, conducted a series of seminars for families whose children care for themselves after school. They used materials developed by the Kansas Committee for the Prevention of Child Abuse: "I'm in Charge."

Working-parent networks. Some companies have ongoing parent groups. Their purpose is to provide continuing information and support. Citibank has such a group. The Financial Women's Association in New York also has a Working Mothers' Committee.

Work and family fairs. COPE in Boston has developed work and family fairs. They are sponsored by a number of businesses and held in or near the workplace. Employees attending the all-day fair have access to a large collection of useful information: books for parents and children, child-care information including summer camps and lists of doctors and dentists who specialize in treating children. Parent-counseling service is also available. The cost to employers is minimal.

Family-centered activities. Opening up the corporation to the families of employees is useful and productive. It gives families an opportunity to learn more about the employees' work and to meet co-workers. These occasions can be festive. Every several years, Merck stages an elaborate family day. Labs, plants, and offices are open for touring. There is food, music, and entertainment for the children.

It becomes evident in detailing family-responsive corporate policies and practices that a great deal of creative thinking has been applied to the solution of work/family problems. Unfortunately, these solutions often exist primarily for the higher strata of the working population, those who work in large corporations or who have upper-level jobs. Though this population is certainly stressed, there is also recourse to other supports. It can only be hoped that family-responsive programs continue to spread to a wider population.

How Corporate Executives Perceive
Work/Family Issues

At a Bank Street luncheon on the changing family that was attended by personnel officers of several corporations, one of the participants posed a question: "There has been a great deal of media coverage about work and family issues," she said. "I read articles in general interest and business magazines, in the lifestyle as well as the financial section of newspapers; I listen to programs on radio and watch them on television. Is it possible—or how could it be possible—that the senior managers of companies don't know that there is an upheaval occurring within their workforce?" At other conferences, similar questions are asked: "What are corporate executives' attitudes about their employees' family needs? Are these attitudes dependent on the executive's age or personal experience—that is, does a manager who has a wife at home differ from a manager who is from a two-career family?"

The Work and Family Life Studies (WFLS), currently being conducted by Bank Street College, have been designed to investigate these and other questions. The Corporate Work and Family Life Study is examining how workers in one high-tech multinational corporation balance their work and family life, identifying which factors are most significantly related to satisfaction on the job and in the marital and parenting relationships. Also, it is identifying those factors most related to stress at home and at work. In this study the workers identify workplace changes that they believe will improve the quality of their family life and their productivity at work. Based on their choices, one change will be agreed upon by the employer and employees and will be implemented.

One of the substudies of the Corporate Study is the Decision-Maker Study (DMS), conducted by me and my colleagues Karen Blum and Richard Ruopp. The DMS was conducted at the corporation that is serving as the site for the corporate WFLS. It is a high-tech multinational company with approximately four thousand workers at this particular site. In this effort, we investigated how the corporate decision makers in one division of the company perceive the work/family issues of their employees; and what the barriers or incentives are to change. The sample for the DMS includes senior officers, vice-presidents, and executive directors of the Research and Development Division, a division containing 1300 people. In addition, senior managers of the Human Resources Division were interviewed. Twenty people, eighteen men and two women, were interviewed. Reported here are preliminary findings.

Each manager was asked the same series of questions. Two DMS staff members were present—one conducting the interview, one taking notes. In addition, all but one of the interviews were tape-recorded and transcribed. The interview lasted approximately forty-five minutes.

At this company, several of the top executives defined committed workers as those who were in the labs early in the morning, late at night, and on the weekends. Some took note of whose cars were in the parking lot during these hours. In my view, it is precisely this attitude that makes the DMS interesting. In some ways, the scientist is the antithesis of the family person. The scientist is expected to be devoted, consumed, to put in very long hours. Virtually all of the executives said, "You can't start an experiment at 8:30 in the morning and know it will be over by 5:00." It is to be noted that, while this company has its own characteristics that have grown out of its history, the commitment expected of workers is not atypical of other corporations.

The Human Resources Division views employees as resources to be developed so that they will be productive both now and in the future. The staff in this company is committed to examining the changing nature of the workforce and developing family-oriented policies. The implementation of flexitime was one of the first efforts toward this goal. Here is one division standing for excellence in science, the other for excellence in employee policies and practices. Let us take a closer look at how and why these complex and somewhat conflicting attitudes are played out.

PRELIMINARY RESULTS

Has the work ethic changed? Working hard was a value to all of the managers we interviewed. Over half, however, felt that people do not work the way they used to. The reasons noted, interestingly enough, were not family-centered: the increased use of van pools for commuting, the growing importance of employees' outside interests, hobbies, or the use of time renovating houses. It was the newcomers, on the rise in the corporate hierarchy, who felt that people were more industrious, more committed than in the past.

What are managers' attitudes toward employed women? This company has made a recent attempt to hire more professional women. There is an affirmative action program in place, with one of its goals to increase the numbers of women in management. The numbers are still small. Several women have reached the top level of middle management; none is yet at the senior vice-president level.

The specter of a woman leaving the job for marriage and children still looms large in some executives' minds. One manager said, "There are a lot of people that feel if you hire women and train them well, they're still going to leave or go on maternity leave. When they come back, they will have lost a lot of the skills they had prior to leaving."

Several managers talked about the practical issues of handling maternity leaves: finding replacements, suspending projects, or picking up the extra work themselves. Even so, most were committed to making this effort for a worker *they valued*, feeling that it is a necessary aspect of retaining competent women. It is clear that any worker, male or female, who makes it known that home is more important than work would not be taken very seriously in this workplace.

One group of managers felt that the increase of women employees was positive. They stated that as managers they did not think about whether the worker was male or female. More important was the employee's capacity to do the job. One woman manager, however, felt it was not that simple. She has come to the conclusion that it is "harder for women to deal with men than for men to deal with men. It isn't because we're uncomfortable, but men have a way of knowing how to react to each other that we don't. We don't know the same set of rules. It's very, very subtle and it's not meant to be discriminatory."

When asked about the role of women at this company, virtually every manager named several women who are "able to have it all and do it all." These women were often referred to as superwomen. One manager spoke about the time when the first of these superwomen was pregnant several years ago. "We'd never had a woman manager pregnant and everyone was wondering how she was going to carry it off. Would she quit? Would she feel comfortable walking around in maternity clothes? She worked all the way to the end and set an example. She came back to work and was more competent than ever." Most of the men managers, in discussing these women, remarked "I don't know how they do it." One felt there were limits to doing it all. He has warned one woman that "she'd better stop having babies if she wants to make vice-president."

What kind of work/family issues do managers face? We asked all the managers: "In your role as vice-president [or other position of interviewee] have you faced any issues related to the work/family needs of your employees—for example, workers having problems with child care or the care of aging parents?" In half the interviews, the managers mentioned women in general and such issues as maternity leave. When asked to specify, they shifted the discussion to male employees with extreme problems such as alcoholism or marital conflicts.

We began to wonder if male employees were more likely to discuss work/family problems with their supervisors than women were. We also wondered if a man or woman in the throes of a problem would be treated differently. Although the men managers tended to deny that there were differences, the two women felt there were. One said that she was afraid she was guilty of being more sympathetic to males than to female employees. The other woman manager said, "I think that perhaps there's a little bit more understanding of men having family problems than women. A lot of managers feel in the back of their minds that when they hire a woman she's going to have problems. They're expecting it. And it was probably initiated by some action on her part. But if a man's having problems, then it's probably genuine."

Let me pause a moment to accentuate these two points:

— Managers may be more aware of the extreme issues and less aware of the everyday issues. In a census at this same company, one third of all the respondents found it "difficult" or "very difficult" to balance work and family life on an everyday basis. This included equal numbers of men and women but was more likely to include employees with young children.
— Managers may be less likely to hear about problems from women than from men.

If this is true, the reasons behind it are complex. It may be simply that this division has more men employees than women. Or it may reflect one phase of a historical change. A decade ago it was hoped that the influx of women into the labor market would bring in feminine values or would "humanize" the workplace. Two recent surveys indicate that, at the present time, managerial women may be more likely to adopt traditional work values than to want to change the workplace toward more family-centered policies. Keller Brown and Kagan (1982) surveyed 1500 managerial women through *Working Woman* magazine. Forty-seven percent of the sample were married; 27 percent had children. The respondents were asked to rate their overall goals. (They could have more than one goal in each rating, from the most to least important.) The results show that "earning more money" was the first goal of 85 percent of the respondents. Surprisingly low on the list were marriage (9th) and family (13th). A survey of 1460 managers for the American Management Association by Schmidt and Posner (1983) found similar results: female managers revealed dramatically stronger career orientations than their male counterparts. In a matched sample, they were more likely to indicate that career rather than home gave them the greater satisfaction. They were also more likely to give up an important family function if it conflicted with work. Similarly, 45 percent of the women as opposed to 31 percent of the men would not turn down a promotion even if it required a change in lifestyle. The influx of women into the workforce and into the managerial ranks is an ongoing process. Much of the impact still remains unknown.

When should the company be involved in developing programs that help workers balance their work and family life? The managers interviewed felt that there was a fine line between appropriate corporate involvement on one hand and interference or paternalism on the other. This line has moved dramatically in the past ten years. As one manager pointed out, "What used to be considered interference is now considered acceptable." There was unanimity that the company's role is to become involved whenever job performance or productivity is affected.

In what ways should the company be involved? The preferred method of corporate involvement in work/family issues was for managers to have the flexibility to solve problems as they arise. One manager voiced this point of view in saying, "I've never had a problem that couldn't be solved by a manager." Several managers noted that there should be company policies to give managers guidelines.

Whereas flexibility of managers is crucially important, there are two problems with a total reliance on this approach:

— There can be difficult personnel relationships that inhibit the effectiveness of managers in solving problems. In the WFLS census, 19.5 percent of the workers in the Research and Development Division indicated that the relationship between supervisor and supervisee, the mood and politics at work, was the aspect of work that most needed changing. It is obvious that some managers are more sensitive than others, so that placing the major initiative for dealing with work/family issues at the manager's discretion is an uneven approach.

— The second problem is the potential of creating a selective system. Those accorded the most tolerance in relation to work/family problems are those employees who are most valued. As numerous managers said, they would bend over backwards for such employees. And in fact there are reported examples such as permitting one woman part-time work as a transition back from maternity leave. Flexibility or sensitivity is less likely to be accorded to employees lower on the status scale.

Which managers are most responsive to work/family issues? At conferences on work and family it is frequently hypothesized that companies will adopt more family-responsive policies when the corporate decision makers are members of two-parent working families. The factors seen as contributing to the sensitivity of managers are age, sex, background, experience, expectations, and values. We found in the Decision-Maker Study that no one of these factors alone seems to be associated with a family-responsive attitude. For example, one manager had an employed wife who had always been granted a great deal of flexibility and compassion by her employer, including a flexible part-time professional job. When asked if such policies would work at his company, the manager replied, "Not here. We're different." It is possible that this man did not have much responsibility for overseeing the housework or child care in his family and that overall responsibility for family work, rather than just the experience of being in a two-parent working family, is a more significant factor in developing sensitivity. But one woman manager, who had a great deal of family responsibility (as well as a great deal of family support), noted that she was less sensitive than others. Because she had made it in the corporate world as it now exists, why shouldn't others? On the other hand, one of the most sensitive managers had no children.

We have concluded that there may be leadership style that is the critical factor. The least sensitive managers were absorbed in their jobs and were less inclined to care about the employees beyond their job performance. One manager remarked, "No one has ever asked me about my family in all the years I've worked here. Therefore I don't ask others." On the other side there were managers who could be characterized, as Peters and Waterman (1983) do in *In Search of Excellence*, as those who "walk around." These managers knew their employees as people, saw them as capable of future growth, and felt they would perform more effectively if they were treated humanely.

INITIAL CONCLUSIONS

The preliminary results of the DMS are provocative. In this division of the company it will probably be some time before the senior management sees work/family issues as salient. Thus it will not be enough for companies to institute family-responsive programs and policies. They must be accompanied by management training. The purpose of the training should be to enlist managers' commitment to the programs, to sensitize them to the concerns of their employees, and to have them share in the development of programs that resolve these problems in ways that fit the company culture.

There are no quick answers, no magic solutions that will work for all employees. Managers will continue to represent many different viewpoints. But a change is occurring, however slowly, and that change might improve life for all concerned: the corporation, the worker, and the worker's family.

8 *

Utilitarianism in the Regulation of Corporate and Family Life

THERE IS OFTEN a fine line between defense and adaptation that parents who work must grapple with both at their workplace and at home. The concept of defense is one of the building blocks of psychoanalytic theory. It helps to explain how individuals maintain psychological equilibrium under the stresses that sometimes originate in external circumstances and sometimes in alterations within the personality. In its early usage, defense referred specifically to the repression of painful ideas and feelings as the means for guarding consciousness against the instrusion of unacceptable material. Observation, along with clarification in theory, led to the broadening of the concept to include an array of mechanisms. Although still important, repression was only one of the variety of protective devices available to the ego.

Even more detailed observation expanded defense in two directions: into the realm of character formation, and into the structures of group formation and social organization that provide defensive functions to augment individual defenses. The mechanisms of defense, along with character as protective armor and membership in established social structures, protect the psyche from the onslaught of either excessive or unacceptable stimuli. But defense exacts costs in exchange for maintaining psychic equilibrium.

The psychic and social costs are implicit in the fact that defenses appear in a hierarchical order corresponding to stages of development. Defenses that appear during later stages of development, such as intellectualization, rationalization, and repression, often limit pleasure but seldom sacrifice the individual's access to reality and rationality. The more primitive defenses, such as denial and projection, are established earlier in development; they distort the individual's perceptions of and attachment to reality. Sacrifices in both pleasure and reality are directly involved in pathological processes. What clinicians look for first in understanding the formation of psychological symptoms is the failure of established defenses. In order to reestablish equilibrium, the psyche resorts to more primitive and hence costly defenses. As Freud pointed out in his famous paper on paranoia, it is a common error to confuse the spontaneous efforts of the mind to cure itself with the underlying illness (Freud, 1911). He suggested that what appear at first blush to be the symptoms of the illness are in fact the regrouping of defenses in order to ward off the more catastrophic illnesses that will occur if psychological deterioration continues. From this brief summary of the theory of defense, it becomes apparent that defense and adaptation are intertwined. Higher-order defenses are adaptive in certain social situations, while primitive defenses sacrifice adaptation to reality for protection against the morbid unraveling of personality structure.

The mechanism of defense called isolation provides an important link that connects the reality of the family and the world of work (Zaleznik, 1979). Isolation is the separation of thinking from feeling. Although it does not occupy the least expensive position in the hierarchy of defenses, it does not stand among the primitive. Isolation is commonly found as a prominent feature in obsessional neurosis, in that the elaboration of thinking prevents individuals from experiencing and understanding how they feel. It is a way of solving the problem of ambivalence in feelings toward other people and particularly prevents aggressive feelings from reaching consciousness.

Isolation of thinking and feeling tends to be highly adaptive in certain situations. It is especially valued in large organizations and often sustains membership, enables career advancement, and promotes job satisfaction. A wide range of emotions, both experienced and expressed, is often unacceptable in the interchanges of people in modern organizations. Generally, the more bureaucratic the organization, the more it rewards isolation and punishes the expression of emotions. If one does not experience emotions, one is less likely to express them. In the more entrepreneurial organizations and in those that place a premium on creativity and innovation, there is greater tolerance of affects and thus less need for isolation on the part of members. The preponderance of large organizations with their bureaucratic cultures overwhelmingly supports isolation. Consequently, the institutions concerned with individual development gear their socialization practices to teach people to separate thinking and feeling. Of course this teaching is not explicit, let alone conscious, in the formation of socialization practices. Indeed, this absence of awareness makes the socialization practices even more powerful than if institutions deliberately set out to foster selected character traits or styles of behavior.

Given the prevalence of isolation as a defense, what are the consequences for the family? Does this defense serve the same adaptive purposes in the family as it does in the dynamics of organizations? These questions have special relevance today because of the increasing prevalence of the two-career family in society. While effects of isolation as a defense tend to be maladaptive for families in general, it is probably highly damaging in the modern two-career family. Isolation limits the ability of parents to enter effectively into the emotional mainstream of family life, with potentially disastrous consequences in raising children. Emotional expression that is both limited and separated from the content of communication within a family threatens the child's sense of identity and conveys a feeling of being disregarded. The net effect is to heighten anxiety.

My purpose in this chapter is to go beyond isolation as a defense and to consider how the forms of thinking and interaction in organizations habituate people to certain stylistic responses in family life. I shall extend the hypothesis that adaptation to these forms in work life becomes maladaptive in family life. This hypothesis is extendable because of the singular importance of power and dependency in both organizations and the family.

Emotion and Utility

In all realms of life, but particularly in organizations, tension exists in the polarization of two major kinds of subjective experiences. One pole is represented in free-floating feelings, perhaps intuitive if not impulsive responses. Charismatic leadership is an example of the more emotional type of management in an organization. At the other extreme of subjective experience is the practice of utilitarianism.

Pure emotion is best understood in loving (or hating) another person, in identifications, and in empathic attachment. Utilitarianism is the calculus of costs and benefits. Sometimes called "trading off," the object of this calculus is to maximize individual net returns. Utilitarianism follows the principle of marginal utility in economic theory. As a normative rule of behavior, individuals should perform certain actions up to the point where the cost of the last increment of behavior equals exactly the incremental reward secured from this behavior. This principle explains much that one observes in the behavior in modern organizations.

The tension between the subjective experience of emotion and utilitarianism plays a part in answering basic questions individuals pose to themselves when they work in organizations. These questions are asked silently and seldom are exposed to the perceptions of other people: (1) To what extent will this organization satisfy my needs? This question involves the problem of *dependency* in organizations. (2) Who are my friends and enemies—on whom can I count to support the activity in which I take an interest? This second question is the *alliance* problem of organizations and involves the ways individuals seek to enhance their position by forming coalitions within the organization. (3) What are the ideals and values I should emulate to enjoy a sense of self-esteem in this organization? This question centers on the problem of *identification* and the elaboration of the individual's ego ideal.

For each of these three questions there is a utilitarian and an emotional mode for providing an answer. In general, the utilitarian mode, involving the cost-benefit calculus, is the primary way in which organizations support individuals in seeking their answers.

Take, for example, the dependency problem: To what extent will this place satisfy my needs? At the purely emotional end of the spectrum, the answer should be "to an unlimited degree." If individuals in fact behaved as if they expected unlimited support, they would soon develop a sense of entitlement about themselves and the organization. There are very few places I know that would countenance this kind of approach. The organization will simply not find it possible to meet such expectations for any length of time. This is not to say that people do not try to cultivate entitlements. The way people preconsciously strive to erect a scaffolding of entitlements is one of the most interesting and subtle aspects of the human side of organizations. But there is a harsh fact to be faced. If the bulk of an organization consisted of people cultivating entitlements, nothing would get done, nothing of economic value would be produced, and in effect the many would be relying on the few to provide for their well-being. It would be inequitable as well as economically untenable.

Examine, however, the other extreme, which is the answer to the dependency problem provided from the utilitarian frame of reference. A peculiar kind of power game arises as the unforeseen consequence of the utilitarian principle. When people cultivate interests at a manifest level, they are also working hard to reverse the dependency flows that arise in power relations. According to the utilitarian model, in situations where an individual may have cause to feel dependent on others, he should try to reverse the flow and make other people dependent on him. The efforts to reverse dependencies produce commonplace yet remarkable kinds of behavior. In its purest form, this behavior requires bargaining in almost every sphere of the individual's activity in the organization.

The utilitarian model provides a normative framework to guide people in negotiating and bargaining: it becomes extremely important not to reveal your hand. You have to be guarded, cautious, and learn to use resources carefully. The calculation of odds must precede any move at any given time. Imagine a life situation in which all of the actors are supreme calculators and, moreover, are trying to disguise the nature of their game. Communication and trust cannot be taken for granted. Above all, people do not (or should not) invest their confidence in other human beings. The extreme position, where the individual successfully has reversed the dependency flow, occurs in situations where he has carefully cultivated options and is prepared to leave the organization unless he gains his goals. From the utilitarian point of view, this means that the operative rule of the game is to withhold commitment. You pack up your intellectual and emotional resources and stand ready to move at the opportune moment. When the potential for mobility becomes understood, your bargaining power increases significantly and is available for use in all situations, particularly where the individual has major economic value.

But there is a particular kind of tyranny to this utilitarian approach. When individuals climb the power ladder, rung by rung, and approach the top, they realize that their ability as calculators has probably helped them to climb. They also believe, though, that the prospects for remaining at the top depend upon their continuing adroitness at calculation in their relations with subordinates. At the extreme these individuals live in fear of being outwitted and humiliated.

In another culture and another time, two principles governed how people should act in a power relationship: an individual should be loyal to his or her organization, and an individual should support the boss. To preserve the integrity of authority, one supported those who legitimately exercised power. In turn, a reciprocal notion applied: it was the job of the power figure to exercise responsibility and fulfill obligations toward others. A boss was supposed to look after the interests of subordinates and make certain that their interest remained uppermost in his or her mind. Authorities therefore sought to exercise power in such a way as to accomplish the purposes of the organization and to support the people involved.

Under conditions of modern power relations, where the utilitarian mode dominates, the ideals of loyalty and obligation, of commitment and fulfillment of expectations, have receded from consciousness. Instead the ideals of independence and of maximizing net returns dominate, which suit the purposes of professionalism and careerism.

From Work to Family

Let us now shift the focus of our attention to the family. When an individual becomes an expert in the utilitarian calculus, there is a strong tendency to apply the same skills or mental habits to the family. I recently overheard a successful man talk about the problems of raising his children. He described his children as amply endowed with intelligence and talent. They did exceedingly well on standardized tests but, according to this distressed father, indicated little interest in working hard. So they were not performing well in school, to the great consternation of their father. His way of handling the problem followed the utilitarian's approach: "If you study for two hours you get to watch television for one." This is a classical example of trading off. With the best of intentions this father was creating a bargaining situation to accomplish the end of getting his children to be what he wanted, which also coincided with his beliefs about their best interests. But the emotional mode was also at play. The use of bargaining appears rational, but it may represent a form of suppressing aggression on the father's part. This suppression would not escape the notice of the children. They learn by identification and similarly use aggression in a passive way. Children learn to irritate their parents by their passivity or lack of responsiveness and gain whatever pleasure this provocation might produce.

Even under the most favorable social and cultural conditions, the utilitarian's approach to the family will falter. As suggested earlier, however, the modern dual-career family presents additional problems. In the traditional family structure, if the working father tried to be the extreme utilitarian and carried his skills from work into the family, there tended to be some counterbalance on the part of the mother, who traditionally accepted responsibility for child care and the home. The mother in this traditional family more than offset the strict utilitarian mode of the father. She also could influence an otherwise stern and calculating father to elicit more direct emotional expression and sensitive reactions. Much, of course, depended upon the closeness of the parents and their basic love and need of each other.

In the more fluid role situations found in the family of the 1980s, both parents do not simply work for a living but follow careers that involve powerful elements of identity and self-esteem. Women pursuing careers discover that, to get along in organizations, they have to become utilitarian and learn to calculate. They and their male partners both become adroit in using these skills in relation to their children and to each other. The end result is a tendency to limit communication and burden the more dependent members of the family with the need to suppress their feelings.

Is there a way out of this dilemma? I have argued that there is a difference between managers and leaders, both in the way they behave and in their psychological makeup (Zaleznik, 1977). Leaders are personally involved in their work and human relationships. Managers tend to be detached utilitarians. Organizations need more leaders and fewer managers, and the same view can be applied to the modern family. This is not a plea to abandon rationality in favor of emotions. Rather it is a suggestion that all institutions in society, including the family, need a model of leadership that is neither purely emotional nor utilitarian but represents some fusion of the two extremes.

Utilitarianism cannot be criticized for its logic. But visualize the kind of leadership that uses emotions to inform utilitarian considerations and a utilitarianism that connects emotions to people and situations more than they usually are. This fusion represents another kind of ideal that I think appears in the best leaders. It is reflected in a person's capacity to communicate directly as well as to understand the nature of symbolism in human relationships. This form of communication contrasts sharply with the signaling, indirection, and guardedness that seem characteristic of bargaining. Indirect communication and signaling often enable people to avoid responsibility for saying what they mean and meaning what they say.

Being a parent is a form of leadership. Though there is nothing new in this idea, it deserves careful consideration. What are the implications of leadership in family life? Individuals who lead in organizations and the family face the psychological task of coming to terms with power. They must be willing to accept the power inherent in their position and be willing to elaborate on it, develop it, and use it. Organizations are hierarchical arrangements just as families are hierarchical arrangements. Parents make a mistake, along with leaders of organizations, when they are unwilling to recognize the power inherent in the positions they occupy and when they are unwilling to use this power.

The father who was bargaining with his children made a false assumption. The children did not need a bargainer—they needed a strong leader. By this I do not mean a figure who is irrational, autocratic, or sadistic. I mean leaders who have the strength of character to stand up for what they believe. If study is an important thing in the household, then the parents will exemplify this by their own approach. And if they view life in the family as managing a complex system or situation, they are going to disturb their children: the parents will be unable to cope with the emotional demands the children are making on them. Their own childhood experience often causes ambivalent feelings in adults when it is their turn to assume authority and responsibility. Ambivalence breeds uncertainty in how the individual should act and differentiate self from objects. It becomes difficult to separate present circumstances and people from the past. Adults under the stress of ambivalent feelings reenact conflicts from childhood and may confuse what was a personal conflict of the past with the attitudes and feelings of their own children.

The problem of ambivalent attitudes toward power goes beyond the questions of identity, of maintaining a separation and consequently the integrity of self and others. The need to defend against the unconscious rage attached to authority figures of the past often leads to exaggerated attempts to be rational. Creating utilitarian models as a means of communication in the family as well as in the work situation serves defensive purposes and emerges from the complex obsessional mechanisms of such defenses as isolation and reaction formation. As I said earlier, obsessional defenses appear adaptive at work, but they cause problems in family life. Even in large organizations questions arise about the adaptive value of obsessional defenses, particularly where the capacity to solve problems requires innovative thinking rather than repetition from the past. Putting aside questions of what modern organizations need from leaders and focusing attention on the family, we can see that the antithesis of utilitarianism is contained in the concept of spontaneity. While I cannot undertake a full exploration of spontaneity here, a few suggestions may point the way to examination of the differences between utilitarian calculation and spontaneity.

The dichotomy is clearly not between rational and irrational behavior. Utilitarianism has a rational base in the concept of marginal utility. Applied to communication among people, however, it tends to be pseudo-rational. When power figures must defend against the unconscious aggression that is inherent in ambivalent feelings toward authority, the obsessional defenses dominate. What may make matters worse is that these defenses are easily rationalized under the banner of utilitarianism, causing guilt reactions in response to the sense of disparity between what individuals actually feel and how they are supposed to think.

It would be a false dichotomy to align utilitarianism with controlled behavior and spontaneity with impulsive behavior. The more important distinction is between coercive control and the sense of being oneself in a situation of inequality in power. Utilitarianism provides strong metaphors for communication. When these metaphors are appropriate, both to the relationship and to the content of the communication, people will find them relatively easy to use. But the metaphors are singularly inappropriate when people are supposed to invest confidence in the situation. Such investment allows for variety in metaphor and in the structure of communication. People may find it possible, even convenient, to experiment. Power relations therefore become more fluid, and the distinction between degrees of power may be constructively blurred for a period of time. In contrast, the underlying aim of coercive control is to maintain power distinctions.

In attempting to examine the relation between work and family, I have relied heavily on concepts that belong to individual psychology, with special emphasis on psychoanalytic psychology. This approach assumes that institutional perspectives on human behavior will not permit a fruitful examination of the meaning of experience to the individual who crosses institutional boundaries almost as a matter of routine. The organization and the family can be separated by an institutional perspective, but much will be lost in understanding how the forms of adaptation in one structure will become a disturbing influence in another.

9 ✳

Supplemental Care
for Young Children

Choosing child-care arrangements to supplement the care provided within the family has become an important new responsibility of parents. In today's economy, far more parents than ever before need to work to support a family. The number has risen steadily and dramatically throughout the 1980s, with the most dramatic rise occurring among mothers of preschool children under the age of six. These numbers change so rapidly that by the time they appear in print, they are out of date. The percentage of mothers of children under age eighteen who are in the labor force increased from 40 percent in 1970 to almost 60 percent in 1983. For married women with children under six, the rate jumped from 30 percent to 50 percent in that period. Today 53 percent of children in two-parent families have working mothers, including more than 46 percent of the children under age six. Most of these working mothers have full-time jobs—62 percent of the working mothers with preschool children and more than 70 percent of those with preschoolers. (Figures from Elizabeth Waldman, quoted in Kamerman, 1983.)

As a matter for public debate in the United States, the daycare issue has been a confused swirl of opinions and elusive facts. At the heart of the issue is a conflict between two major functions of families: (1) the economic responsibility to work, to support family members, and to maintain family autonomy, and (2) the responsibility to care for the physical and psychological needs of children in a stable and nurturing environment. The problem of reconciling these responsibilities has often been an agonizing one for millions of American families. Similarly, at the level of public policy, both decision makers and professionals have struggled to define an appropriate role for the community with respect to these family functions.

More than one member of a family now needs to work, since only one in five full-time jobs will support a family of four at a modest budget level. Family income for most families with children achieves the median only because there are two wages. Parents must search for an arrangement for their children during the hours when they have to work, just as they must find basic health and other needed services. The tasks of parenthood have not diminished, but they are different today.

Parents need to perceive themselves as controlling these family functions rather than having no choices or having choices made for them. Yet parents are not responsible for creating the child-care options from which to choose, any more than they are responsible for building hospitals and health centers. Like parents throughout other periods of history and in all cultures, they need the support of a caring community. American parents seldom find it.

If we want strong families to nurture America's children, we should not feel complacent about making the statement that parents feel anxiety and guilt as they place their children in daycare. These are not healthy emotional states. Grief at separation, or fear, would be a strong feeling, but not necessarily destructive; anxiety and guilt are destructive. There is no reason why parents who work hard at a job to support a family, who nurture children during the hours at home, and who have searched for and selected the best arrangement possible for their children should need to feel anxious and guilty. It almost seems as if our culture wants parents to experience these negative feelings.

The Child-Care Trilemma

The issue today is not whether parents should work; they are working and they need to work. Nor is the issue whether child care is good or bad for young children; there is ample evidence that good care is good for children and bad care is bad for them. The real policy issue for working parents can be described as the child-care trilemma.

The first point on the trilemma is quality for children. Most people believe that quality entails, among other things, a fairly low child:staff ratio so that staff can respond to children as individuals. The second point on the trilemma is wages for staff. The third point is affordability for parents.

Since ratios and wages affect costs, the three points to the trilemma are highly interrelated. At present, if any two of the points are arranged satisfactorily, the third point becomes hopelessly unsatisfactory. If wages and ratios are set to accomplish reasonable goals, then the cost of the service goes far beyond what parents can afford. If affordability and wages are satisfactory, quality disappears. If affordability and quality are achieved, wages become so low that staff will not stay in the field. In fact, of the three points to the trilemma, it is wages that have been traded off: child care is now subsidized by caregivers who accept wages far lower than the value of their work (Ruopp et al., 1979; Project Connections, 1981).

The Supply, Visible and Invisible

Parents at present are selecting a wide diversity of arrangements for the care of their children (Rhodes and Moore, 1976; U.S. Census Bureau, 1982). Often they make several arrangements for one child to cover their work hours, and they also must make arrangements for all their children.

Generally, the two major classifications of types of care from which parents select their package of arrangements are care within the family and care in the community (the daycare market).

Care within the family. Care within the family includes all arrangements that parents are able to make with family members in their own households or in the households of relatives and close friends. They include: a parent on parental leave from work; a parent working at home; parents staggering work hours so that someone will be home; an older child caring for a younger sibling; a relative or close friend caring for the child, either in the child's home or the relative's or friend's home; the child caring for himself. Except for the last category, the arrangements listed above have been called "care by kith and kin." Not all parents have such options. About half of all working parents are able to make such an arrangement.

Families that have resources within the family often use them out of preference, not just because they may be free or of low cost (Moore, 1980). While some analysts (Hofferth, 1979) predict that the availability of care by relatives will decline as economic conditions force them into the labor force along with everybody else, this change has not occurred yet. (Rhodes and Moore, 1976; Census Bureau, 1982). Parents who are using care outside the family do not have acceptable available care by kith and kin. There are also data indicating that parents will not be attracted away from in-family types of arrangements, even by high-quality free care in the community (Wiener, 1978).

Care by relatives is different in nature from market child care. Kith and kin have an irrational attachment to a child and the parents that makes this form of care a loving and often unmonetized gift. It should not be romanticized, however. No parent should be forced by the lack of community options to use a relative who is incapacitated, alcoholic, abusive, or sexually deviant, to give examples of the horror stories so well known in the child-welfare field. School-aged children should not have to drop out of school to care for younger children. Like every other form of care, care within the family can be either very good or very bad.

There are at least 1.6 million school-age children caring for themselves, the so-called latchkey children. Reportedly, 99 percent of all parents believe that seven-year-olds should not be left home alone, although many of the same parents have no alternative but to do just that (Whitbread, 1979). Parents leave their young children alone when there is no acceptable arrangement they can afford. As children grow older, parents become less willing to sacrifice other important household budget needs for daycare. The children, too, need more freedom to participate in community activities and will reject poorly designed programs that are not appropriate for their age. For these reasons, most latchkey children are school-age children. Nevertheless, there are also an estimated 20,000 preschool children being left alone while their parents work to support their families (Kennedy, 1982).

Care in the community. The broad category of care in the community covers all the arrangements that parents make when they must find care beyond their family and close friends. These parents are in the child-care market.

The options available to them are many and include the same group programs used by parents who do not work. For three- to five-year-olds in particular, American parents widely use group programs because they perceive that their children need social experiences with peers and opportunities for learning beyond what the single-family household usually can offer. Of this preschool group of children, 64 percent are in some kind of group program, regardless of whether the parents work (Kamerman and Kahn, 1981). It is natural that working parents also turn to these programs, particularly those with a reputation for quality.

Arrangements that working parents may make for their children in the community include the following:

— providers of care in the child's own home, often called "babysitters"
— shared care, or a provider who cares for children of several families in one of the children's homes or rotates to several homes, with parents sharing the cost
— family daycare (definitions vary by states, but usually care of six or fewer children in the caregiver's home)
— group homes (usually six to twelve children in the home of the caregiver, with more than one caregiver to meet ratio requirements)
— center care, including Head Start, nursery schools, and full-day centers and those with extended days, for infants, preschool children, or school-age children before or after school and during vacations

A typology of care in the community has three major dimensions. The first is the type of care as described above, which can be simplified into the categories of center care, family daycare, and care in the child's own home, called in-home care. The second dimension categorizes differences among the children cared for: infants and toddlers; preschool children; school-age children; mixed ages; and children with special needs or family problems. The third dimension is hours of care. Each of these types of care could be offered on a full-day basis or on a part-day basis.

Because of the complexity of these classifications, and because parents may combine several types of care to cover a day even for the same child, the research on use of care has been somewhat confusing. Based on a national consumer study (Rhodes and Moore, 1976), children under the age of fourteen, in care for more than ten hours a week in 1975, were being cared for as follows:

Relative care	5,118,000
In-home care	1,863,000
Family daycare	2,320,000
Center, full- and part-day	2,316,000
Total children	11,617,000

Problems with the Supply

The present child-care system has the advantage of offering parents a variety of options. The problems in the system are: (1) parents need more information about choosing a high-quality arrangement; (2) the cost may be greater than parents can afford; (3) much of the care is hard to find; and (4) the issue of care for children when they are mildly ill is not resolved.

THE FIRST PROBLEM: QUALITY

All the forms of care in the community would be very high or very low in quality. We know from a great deal of research in child care that there are factors that do make a measurable difference in children's test scores and in their behavior. Some of the factors that have been found important to quality are the following:

Group size. A national study found that the overall size of the group of children has a powerful effect on children. Small groups work better (Ruopp et al., 1979). For three- to five-year-olds, when the size of the group is much over 20, quality suffers. Infants need much smaller groups.

Ratios. Child:staff ratios are very important for infant/toddler care. For three- to five-year-olds, they should be half the size of the group (Ruopp et al., 1979).

Staff training. Studies have found that training in child-related topics is important to quality, both for centers and family daycare. For centers, it is also more effective if staff members are trained in the goals and philosophy of the program (Ruopp et al., 1979; Lazar, 1978; Fosberg, 1980).

Educational philosophy. While there is no strong evidence that any particular curriculum is more effective with young children than another, studies have found that programs with a commitment to some goals and educational philosophy are more effective (Lazar, 1978).

Parents' role. When parents and staff work closely together and communicate, children are more successful (Shipman, 1976; Fein, 1979).

Health. Research has found that parents place high priority on health aspects of daycare programs (Rhodes and Moore, 1976). The ideal health program would include training for the staff in detection of problems, appropriate referral services, and emergency and safety procedures; referral and follow-up relationships between the daycare program and health-care professionals in the community; and health education for children, parents, and staff (Richmond and Janis, 1982). The effects of such services have been documented in Health Start and Head Start (Vogt et al., 1973). Attention to health is important not only to the families using the care but to the community at large. Studies have found that frequency of handwashing reduces the number of illnesses and therefore reduces the spread of disease throughout the community.

Features of the environment. Studies in Pasadena (Prescott and Jones, 1967 and 1972) have found that quality for children is associated with the following characteristics:

— daring with safety: children need opportunities to test new skills and explore new things, handling potentially dangerous activities in a safe way
— softness: children need a variety of soft toys, pillows, rugs, gooey materials, adult laps, and other tactile experiences
— variety of activities: children need a range of activities, some of them open-ended with no right way to do them, others offering the challenge of mastering something the right way
— props for dramatic play: make-believe is the use of symbols in fantasy play; props, costumes, and toys that encourage children to act out roles are very important to growth and learning
— clarity: the environment and the materials in it should be organized so that children know where things can be found and what is and is not permitted

— privacy: children need small places where they can withdraw from the group if they want to
— diversity of adults: children benefit from knowing adults
of different ages, different work roles, different sexes, and
different cultures
— affection

The layout of the available space also affects children's behavior.
Large undivided spaces lead to loud and aggressive behavior; smaller
areas where two to six children can work or play together brings
about friendly and cooperative play (Prescott and David, 1979).
The match of program to a child's needs is important as well.
Different children thrive under different conditions, and it is important that there be a variety of options from which parents can
choose the best arrangement for their family (Clarke-Stewart, 1978).

Parents may assume that they will find these qualities in daycare, particularly when it is regulated by the states. There is excellent child care in most communities, so they may indeed find
care with all of the above features. State licensing, however, will
not guarantee this kind of quality (Morgan, 1984). In the first place,
not all child care is covered by licensing. In the case of centers,
some states license only full-day centers and do not regulate part-
day nursery schools. Some states exempt church-run centers. Daycare and preschool programs run by the public schools are not
regulated through licensing because they fall under the jurisdiction
of departments of education and local school officials. In many
communities, school-run daycare is not required by school officials
to meet the standards that private programs must meet.

Family daycare is not regulated at all in some states. It may be
defined in such a way that homes with just a few children do not
meet the definition and do not need to be licensed. Many states
define family day care as three or more children or four or more
children. One state defines it as the care of children from four
different families. Obviously much family daycare is not covered
by these regulatory definitions. In-home daycare is not regulated
except in a few states that monitor providers who are paid with
public funds.

Even in states where coverage of center care and family daycare
is complete, licensing offers a baseline protection that does not
cover all the factors known to be associated with quality. No state

regulates everything in the list given above of research findings about elements of quality. Yet each of these elements is regulated by one or more states. Even if the element is regulated, the state may not be able to require high quality. Licensing sets a level that all providers must meet. For example, ratios in a state are set not at an ideal level but on a level agreed to as feasible. Many providers will go beyond the basic required level to higher levels of quality. Parents will need help from their community in thinking about and in choosing a good arrangement.

Up until now, this discussion has focused on high quality. It is important to remember that there are a few horror stories in child care, even though such occurrences are rare. Children have been physically and sexually abused in daycare in all its forms. Abuse is difficult to regulate: such behavior in adults is so far from social norms as to be abnormal, and of course it is defined by law as criminal behavior. Licensors could not discover it on routine visits, since the adults would behave well when licensors are there. Many states are instituting criminal checks on new daycare center staff and on applicants for family daycare licenses or registration. If these new laws or regulations are implemented, which would be costly in staff time, they will help to weed out a few known offenders. But people who have never been convicted of harming children will not be found in this way.

The best protection parents can have against the nightmare of a daycare arrangement where someone might hurt their child is to choose a place that encourages parents to drop in at any time and that facilitates communication among parents using the program. If parents are free to drop in and if they exercise this right, it is not likely that adults in that place are behaving in ways that harm children. This is a regulatory issue, since many states do guarantee parents this right of access. Those states that do not will probably add this provision to their regulations when the time comes to revise them.

Parents should also listen to their children's reports of what happens in daycare and be alert to behavioral clues. There may be many reasons why a child becomes fearful, hesitant to go off to daycare or clinging to parents. Abuse at the daycare program is almost never the reason, but there is always the remote possibility that it could be. Parents can investigate this by talking to one another to find out what the other children are expressing. Most daycare providers, regardless of the form of care, are dedicated to their work and respect the children in their care. They deserve to have the community protect them by action to screen out unscrupulous and deviant adults. Neither children nor good providers will be protected unless parents, who see their own children and the caregivers every day, pay close attention to the clues they get and to their own perceptions.

THE SECOND PROBLEM: COSTS

The difference between high-quality care and very bad care is actually small, since the initial cost for any care at all is high. Child care is the fourth largest expense of parents, after housing, food, and taxes. Care is expensive since staff must be paid at least a subsistence wage, even if they are untrained (the cost of training may add only a small amount to the cost). Ratios are the one element of quality that strongly affects costs. If child:staff ratios are high, the costs will be lower, since costs vary directly with ratios. Wages of course would affect costs and are important to quality, but wages are generally low right now.

When ratios are low, as in the case of an infant:staff ratio of 3:1 or 4:1, both affordability and wages are affected. Either three or four families of those infants must pay out of their own annual pay enough to support a staff person's full wage for a year. For most parents, that presents a hardship unless they earn a great deal more than the caregiver. If they earn the same, they will have to pay a third to a quarter of their income just to support that caregiver wage, not including the other expenses of the program.

Most parents who are at, just above, or just below the median income cannot afford to pay more than 10 percent of their total family income for the care of all their children (Preschool, 1980). Parents typically pay much more than that for the care of infants, because of their vulnerability and the importance of this period. Parents of school-age children typically are not willing to spend as much as 10 percent of total family income on child care, because of their perception of children's growing independence and the pressures of other important expenses.

When family income is as low as half the median income, parents cannot possibly pay as much as 10 percent of it for child care.

Housing, food, and taxes will have eaten most of their income, and there will be little left for child care. When family income is twice the median, parents probably could pay 10 percent more easily, or even 20 percent, but they are unlikely to want to pay more than 10 percent except for infant care.

Costs vary greatly from one part of the country to another. It is not unusual for infant care to cost $5000, and in some places it can go considerably higher. Preschool care is less, but $3500 is not an uncommon price for a quality arrangement. These are examples of fairly high prices, but very reasonable costs per child in the daycare budget. Parents who can afford to pay $3500 or $5000 will probably be earning $35,000 or $50,000, incomes in the top 10 percent of the population. The median income is around $22,000. Parents at that level can pay about $2200 for the care of all their children. This is not enough to pay for a good child:staff ratio without exploiting staff with low wages. We have traded off wages for quality and affordability.

The largest subsidy for child care is the federal 20-30 percent sliding tax credit on parents' personal income tax. The concept of a sliding credit is a useful one, since parents earning half the median will not benefit as much as parents earning twice the median because they cannot pay as much for child care—the slide makes the credit more equitable. Yet, 30 percent is not enough for a family at half the median income to enable them to choose a quality arrangement. For them, the credit would need to slide at least up to 50 percent. Other forms of subsidy are the Social Services Block Grant, some school programs, and some job-training and employment programs.

THE THIRD PROBLEM: INVISIBLE SUPPLY

Child care is difficult for parents to find even if they have a clear idea of how to look for quality and even if they have no problem with affordability. Much of the supply is invisible because of vagaries in state licensing coverage, and because of the high number of children in family daycare and in-home care. Family daycare providers may not be licensed even if covered by the licensing law, since they may not know about the requirement of licensing. In-home providers are not regulated. Most parents have difficulty finding out what types of care are available and in locating providers.

THE FOURTH PROBLEM: CARE FOR SICK CHILDREN

When parents work, their employers expect them to be on the job for a specified number of days, with vacation time, sick leave, and personal days spelled out. Young children typically have between six and eight respiratory illnesses each year, most of them minor, and one or two digestive illnesses (Aronson, 1984). Children in daycare have a similar number of respiratory illnesses but considerably more gastrointestinal illnesses. The rate of the gastrointestinal illnesses can be dramatically decreased in centers with strict handwashing practices, but young children under the best of conditions are often mildly ill.

Of course, when children are seriously ill, or when an illness is just beginning and it is hard to predict its seriousness, parents will want to be at home with their children. Part of the solution to this issue will have to be more liberal leave policies for parent/employees to care for sick family members. Being at home for all the normal illnesses of young children, however, could easily entail twenty or more days of absence from work in addition to the absences already permitted. This many missed days goes beyond the sick leave and personal days traditionally permitted to working adults. Minor childhood illnesses therefore tend to cause a high degree of anxiety. Working parents believe their children are ill more often than the children of nonworking parents. They tend to call their doctors more often because of their work-related worry, and the doctors too may believe these children are ill more often because of the greater frequency of calls.

Working parents with a stable child-care arrangement usually know that their child will be excluded from care if any symptoms of illness appear. Daycare centers in the past have placed heavy reliance on the exclusion of sick children from care as the primary means of preventing the spread of disease. Most states require centers, and often family daycare as well, to exclude sick children at the first appearance of any symptoms (Johnson, 1983). Centers and states have developed these policies because they believe that children need to be with a parent when they are ill.

There are two problems with this reliance on exclusion. First, children have already spread infectious disease before the first appearance of a symptom. Second, the reliance on exclusion may cause daycare people to neglect other, more useful policies that would inhibit spreading disease, with or without the exclusion policy. One of these useful policies would be staff education in hand-washing procedures. Most daycare staff are aware of the importance of cleanliness, but they do not know how to wash their hands. Training materials, posted procedures, more specific regulations, all are important for daycare.

Exclusion has a side effect on the quality of care for children. Parents and staff develop tensions over a problem that neither alone can solve. The staff blame parents for bringing the child when symptoms of disease appear in the middle of the morning. Parents blame staff because the child is sick so often. Conflict between parents and staff undermine the quality of daycare for children. More recently, public health professionals have begun to become concerned over the exclusion policy because parents may be forced to remove their child from the group already exposed to an illness and take the child somewhere else, where another group of people may be exposed to the infection.

In the last few years there have been several models at the community level for experimenting with ways of caring for mildly sick children (Mohlabane, 1984). Some of the models are:

— training a corps of in-home providers who go to the child's home and receive back-up from their agency
— setting up an infirmary
— listing family daycare providers willing to take in sick children and make provision for them; make the list available to parents
— a satellite family daycare home used by a center for sick children
— hiring additional staff to float, at one or more centers, who can go to a sick child's home and stay with him there
— a get-well room in the child's regular center

Some of these ideas are more workable than others. They will continue to develop in the years to come and will need guidance from health professionals.

Resources and Referral Centers

The above discussion has identified some major problems with the daycare supply. In response to some of these problems, there has been a spontaneous growth of child-care resource and referral centers for parents in different parts of the country (Levine, 1982). In 1972, in Cambridge, Massachusetts, and in the Bay Area of San Francisco, two different daycare services for parents started, performing much the same function but unconnected to one another. In Cambridge, the service was called the Child Care Resource Center; in San Francisco it was called Switchboard. Several other pioneers began similar services soon afterward. For example, in Oakland, California, a service called Bananas was begun because, it was said, parents were going "bananas" trying to solve their daycare problems.

When these resource and referral services were studied in 1979-1982 (Project Connections), only a handful of these R&Rs had developed nationally. More recently, however, there has been a spurt of growth. Employers are beginning to purchase R&R services for their employees. California has funded a network of such services in every area of the state. A few other states, like North Carolina and New Mexico, have funded some demonstrations. Other states and other employers are discussing further support for the R&R functions.

Resource and referral organizations are not information-retrieval services (Morgan, 1980). They play an active role in the supply-demand picture in the daycare market, providing services for parents, providers, and the community. The functions they perform vary, depending on what already exists in the community, since they tend to build on rather than duplicate existing services. But the functions are remarkably similar from one place to another on the whole.

R&Rs compile detailed information on all types of child care, far beyond the licensed lists. They have listings of providers not required to be licensed, and they gather information on vacancies and policies of interest to parents. With these data they are aware of gaps in services, and they tend to stimulate new supply where it is needed, even recruiting family daycare and helping through the licensing processes.

They provide detailed counseling to parents on how to choose a high-quality arrangement that meets their individual needs. They tend to offer or to stimulate training for providers in order to help them better meet the needs and desires of parents. For example, even in communities where there is training for daycare providers, the R&R might begin to offer a type of training that does not exist, such as training in sensitivity to the values of particular cultures. They become a resource for information and training for family daycare providers who would otherwise be isolated, or they put family daycare providers in touch with other resources and help them develop their own organizations with their own resources.

The R&Rs have the only useful data on supply and demand in a particular community. Their supply data are a resource file, which they continually augment and update. Their demand data are a count of actual calls from some of the parents in the community, usually those having trouble matching up with supply. It represents active, effective demand rather than hypothetical need and is useful in shedding light on whether there is unmet demand for particular types of care or care in particular locations.

Because the R&Rs have a working relationship both with parents and with providers, they offer an avenue for relations between health professionals and both these groups for the further improvement of child care.

Conclusions

Today's working families lack a support system in the community. They are confused by conflicting advice, lack of information, and societal ambivalence. It is hard to conceive of any other culture in history that has left its parents so isolated and cut off from a caring community. High-quality care services offer the support of other parents and staff. With such support, parents are helped in their own adult development as generative nurturing parents. Poor child care, however, offers none of these benefits and may be harmful to children.

Fortunately, there are many high-quality arrangements that parents can make in the community, though they are often hard to find and afford. The addition of child-care resource and referral services to the daycare market serves as an active clearinghouse function between supply and demand. It also provides a vehicle for public and private subsidy, and an avenue through which professionals interested in child growth and parent growth can reach both parents and providers for further improvement of the system.

IV *

Special Stresses

*

_____

THE FAMILY'S ABILITY to meet a major internal stress will be quite different from its ability to meet a stress coming from outside. In the face of some societal stress, the family can be seen as a unit pulling together. In the face of internal stress, such as divorce, the forces of grief, isolation, self-incrimination, and anger can be overwhelming. Each individual fights for a kind of personal survival. Parents who are at odds with each other not only cannot support the child in his own struggles but often unconsciously use him as a pawn between them. Acute stresses are likely to cause serious setbacks to his developmental progress, and work by Wallerstein, Camara, and Hetherington (summarized in Kathleen Camara's chapter here) shows that a child's development may be impaired for as much as five years. Since 58 percent of our children will have lived in a single-parent family for a major part of their lives by the time they are eighteen, we are talking about over half of the children in the United States. Camara's chapter addresses some of the effects of divorce, particularly how parental communication that supports a child's developmental needs enables children to cope better with family breakup.

Chronic illness in one family member is bound to have an impact on the rest of the family. How the structure of the family is changed to meet this stress, how outside resources are utilized, as well as the immediate and long-term effects on the family and on each member, need to be understood and assessed. If we can visualize the contemporary responses as symptomatic of regression and reorganization in order to cope, and when we can foresee the long-term effects of such reorganization, we can begin to clarify the roles of professionals in supporting a chronically stressed family system and each of its individuals. John Leventhal and Barbara Sabbeth describe the special stresses of chronic illness and the impact on interpersonal relations with siblings and parents as well as on the sick child and on family resources. They point out the need for effective supports both to develop the child's relatedness to others and to expand the child's opportunities for autonomy.

School-age pregnancy is seen as a failure, and often a hopeless one, for the teenage mother, her child-to-be, and her family. Services for teenage fathers in these situations have been all but ignored; this lack of educational and social support for paternal roles leaves these fathers uninformed about infant care and needs, and perpetuates the problem. Society's strong disapproval and nonsupport at such a time lead to a failure in nurturing these young people in their own development. Lest we see this failure repeated in the infants, we must begin to look more clearly at the stresses on teenage parents and find more positive techniques to help them in parenting. Lorraine Klerman recommends specific measures to ameliorate the adverse impact of both the stress of isolation and the frequent loss of educational opportunity for teenage parents. Studies point up one fact: if the teenage mother can be taken back into her family, her own and her baby's ultimate development will be significantly better. If we hope to break the cycle of poverty and failed achievement for these children and their teenage parents, we must identify the forces at work—familial and societal—and come up with remedies to create better outcomes for both generations.

10 ✳

Family Adaptation
to Divorce

THE HIGH RATES of marital dissolution and the increase in the numbers of single-parent households in the United States present complex challenges to American family life. With nearly half of the marriages formed in the 1970s expected to end in divorce (Cherlin, 1981), and with a large percentage of these divorces occurring in families with children under eighteen years of age, an increasing number of parents and children can be expected to experience substantial changes in their family lives. For some families, the changes accompanying divorce will result in prolonged physical, psychological, and social distress; other families may develop methods of adapting that will allow them to adjust more easily. The variability in family reponses suggests that investigations of the long-term effects of divorce must include a study of the conditions that support healthy transitions to changed family forms, roles, and functions.

Studies of healthy adaptations to stressful life events typically use a stress and coping framework. Most research in this area applies theories of stress and coping to the adjustment of individual family members to life events. This perspective needs to be expanded to account for the adjustment that is required in group patterns of interaction among family members. As Reiss (1981) suggests, the study of individual coping strategies may yield a different picture from one that focuses on family strategies. Systems theory views changes in family life as developmental transitions that offer opportunities for positive adjustment on the part of the family as a whole. Thus the total family system (including individuals and subsystems within the family) becomes the unit of analysis for the examination of adaptation to a stressful life event. In this chapter I use a systems approach to review the processes and factors associated with the successful adaptation by parents and children to changes accompanying divorce.

The Experience of Divorce

Coping with divorce involves managing a complex array of conditions and changes. Patterns of interaction among family members change with the transition from a two-parent to a one-parent household. Family members must develop and adjust to new routines, schedules, and living arrangements. Financial resources, redistributed to support two households, are diminished, and families may be required to relocate to less expensive housing. Changes in residence may result in the loss of social supports for adults and children. The economic pressures may require parents to assume additional work outside the home, thereby reducing the amount of time that parents can give to children (Weitzman, 1981).

The substantial changes in living conditions and relationships are accompanied by, and may further exacerbate, existing emotional strains. These strains are seen in a wide range of emotional reactions displayed by both parents and children over very short periods; emotions ranging from relief and euphoria to ambivalence and uncertainty, bitterness, anger, hostility, and depression (Weiss, 1975). The emotional, financial, and social stresses of divorce may lead to the development of psychological disturbances, as documented in the longitudinal studies of Hetherington, Cox, and Cox (1982) and Wallerstein and Kelly (1980). Several comprehensive reviews of studies of the effects of divorce are available (see Bloom, Asher, and White, 1978; Camara, Baker, and Dayton, 1980; Hetherington and Camara, 1984; Hetherington, Camara, and Featherman, 1982; Kitson and Raschke, 1981; Shinn, 1978).

However, researchers and reviewers of research in this area have noted the variations that exist within the groups of divorced families studied. Husbands, wives, and children within the same family system may assess their experiences of divorce very differently (Barnard, 1972; Camara, 1979; Levinger, 1966; Weiss, 1975). While some families appear to adjust more easily to the life changes associated with divorce, others experience prolonged psychological, social, and economic stress (Bloom, Asher, and White, 1981; Hetherington, Cox, and Cox, 1982; Kitson and Rashcke, 1981). Recent studies have identified factors that account for some of the variations occurring in post-divorce families. These factors are related to current theories of stress and family functioning.

THEORIES OF STRESS AND FAMILY FUNCTIONING

System theorists view the family as an organized whole, so that elements within the system are necessarily interdependent. As described by Minuchin (1985), the system is characterized by circular patterns of causality and by homeostatic features that maintain the stability of functioning patterns. Interactions among family members are defined by family rules, cohesion, affective involvement, communication, and role boundaries. When divorce occurs, these patterns are upset, affecting all members of the family. In order to restore equilibrium, existing patterns and the behaviors of all members of the family system must change.

"Coping" refers to this complex process of change whereby individuals respond to a stressful event by acquiring and using their resources to adjust to the demands of a situation. Thus to cope means to counteract the effects of stress in an attempt to restore equilibrium. The ability of the family to respond to the demands of a stressful event can be assessed along four dimensions: timing, the presence of additional stressors, the availability of personal, family, and social supports, and characteristics of individual family members. These dimensions predict whether existing patterns of interaction will be altered in ways that will either help the family system achieve a new equilibrium or that will maintain a dysfunctional interactional pattern within the family.

First, divorce represents a process of change rather than a discrete event. The point during the process at which families are studied dictates the nature and degree of impact of divorce on family members. When stable patterns of functioning are no longer adequate to deal with stress, the system must reorganize (Minuchin,

1985). Reorganization takes time, and the family may have to endure transitional adjustments before it can effectively organize its resources to accommodate to the new situation. When this occurs, the transition to healthy adjustment may be mislabeled as pathological (Walsh, 1982). For example, the time of separation of parents appears to be the most stressful for adults and children (Hetherington, Cox, and Cox, 1979; Wallerstein and Kelly, 1980).

Second, if divorce is complicated by continuing unresolved pressures and ongoing hardships, most family members will have trouble adapting to the changes in their lives. Some of the stresses leading to difficulties in adjustment include continuing conflict between former spouses; forced maternal employment and increased unavailability of parents to children; social isolation; psychological disturbance or substance abuse in parents; and increased financial pressures coupled with decreased financial resources (Brown, 1976; Coletta, 1979; Hess and Camara, 1979; Hetherington, Cox, and Cox, 1982). Families facing these stressors tend to increase the rigidity of their interactional patterns, are unable to maintain clear role boundaries, and may avoid or resist exploration of alternative interactional patterns. Thus these families become stuck in dysfunctional patterns of interaction that may maintain or exacerbate the stresses with which they are confronted.

Third, the resources that families are able to marshall to reduce stress will predict the degree of their adjustment to divorce. Internal and external resources provide the additional energy the family requires in times of stress so that adaptable patterns of functioning may emerge (Walsh, 1982). The family can be aided by personal resources, family resources present before the divorce, and social supports. Personal resources include finances, education, good health, and psychological support (George, 1980). Predivorce family resources consist of cohesion, adaptability, communication, and problem-solving skills (Burr, 1973). Social supports typically come from kin, neighbors, friends, or self-help groups for parents and children.

Finally, the form and effectiveness of responses to a stressful event may be modified by age, level of development, sex, and genetic factors (Dunn, Kendrick, and McNamee, 1981; Hess and Camara, 1979; Hetherington, 1981; Rutter, 1983; Wallerstein and Kelly, 1980). The coping patterns of children of different ages and developmental levels are not the same. (These are described in a later section of this chapter.) Boys, compared to girls, appear to be more vulnerable to the variety of life stresses. In addition, genetic factors may operate so as to render some persons more vulnerable to environmental influences.

The assessment of the effectiveness of particular coping strategies remains a complex problem. What may be an effective strategy for one person within the family system may not work for another in another system. Furthermore, what may be effective at one point during the process of adjustment may not be helpful at another point. For example, while alignment with one parent against the other may serve a child's immediate needs for security, this strategy may be dysfunctional in the long run. Obtaining a second job may result in decreased financial strain for parents but may contribute to increased loneliness and frustration for children.

Overall, it would appear that successful coping depends on the flexibility, adaptability, and availability of a range of strategies in response to a stressful event, each of which is associated with the timing or "pile up" of additional stressors, availability of personal, family, and social resources, and such individual characteristics as age, developmental level, sex, and genetic disposition. Yet in order for the family system to achieve new levels of equilibrium following the initial post-divorce period, a number of factors associated with healthy adjustment must be present.

Healthy Post-Divorce Adjustments

Recent studies of the post-divorce family have identified several conditions related to the positive functioning of adults, children, and family systems after divorce (Ahrons, 1980; Camara, 1985; Hess and Camara, 1979; Hetherington, Cox, and Cox, 1979; Kalter, 1977; Wallerstein and Kelly, 1980). The factors that seem most predictive of positive outcomes following divorce include reduction of conflict; maintenance of close relationships with children; provision of a secure and predictable environment; flexibility and adaptability of parents in redefining roles; and the availability of social support. It should be noted that the results presented here are based largely on studies of white, middle-income family samples. Little research to date has examined the coping mechanisms and adjustment patterns used by lower-income families and by those of black or Hispanic origin.

REDUCING CONFLICT

To the extent that parents are able to reduce their overt conflict, children will adjust more easily to the divorce. When conflict is minimized, children exhibit less aggression and fewer social problems in their play with peers, fewer symptoms of disturbance such as withdrawal or acting out, more effective study and work behaviors at school, and better overall functioning (Hess and Camara, 1979; Wallerstein and Kelly, 1980).

For most families, the period surrounding the actual separation and divorce is marked by conflict and acrimony. In some cases, conflict between spouses may become even more intense following separation. Ahrons (1980) suggests that the absence of rules defining how and when each of the parents should continue to relate to children creates much of the confusion and stress experienced by family members. She explains that the lack of role models and the absence of societal norms for developing a continuing relationship between divorced parents complicate the transition to a divorced coparenting relationship. Adults who find that they are able to function effectively in their post-divorce parenthood roles identify flexibility, compromise, and the willingness to accommodate to each other's needs and schedules as important factors. Parents who recognize the importance of their child's relationship with the other parent can make active attempts to reduce or contain their conflict (Camara, 1985).

Where acrimony between former spouses has not abated, more formal schedules and agreements may be required to reduce instances of overt conflict. In these situations, the spouses can still maintain a moderate level of interparental cooperation if they center their relationship on child-related concerns. Formal schedules and agreements may enable former spouses to deal with each other in predictable ways, which focus on their joint responsibilities for caretaking of children and which may prevent interactions from spilling over into conflict-ridden domains.

To illustrate the coping mechanisms used by spouses in high-conflict families, several examples from families involved in my current research study will be used (Camara, 1985). In families where there are high levels of conflict and high levels of cooperation around issues related to childrearing, parents develop mutually acceptable, formalized schedules for transferring children from one household to another. These parents set aside times when children are not present to discuss problems and may agree to avoid discussions of topics that are either too sensitive or not directly related to the post-divorce family situation. In addition, these parents separate adult issues from child-centered parental concerns. In cases where even minimum levels of communication are not possible, the former spouses limit contact to short, predetermined, and scheduled conversations. Despite the existence of continued anger one spouse may feel toward the other, parents in these families attempt to develop a working coparental relationship that acknowledges the importance of both parents in the child's life, and attempts to reduce the amount of stress engendered when there is continuing overt conflict.

MAINTAINING CLOSENESS WITH CHILDREN

Even in families where spouses cannot contain their conflicts in order to cooperate, parents may be able to cushion some of the negative effects by maintaining close individual relationships with their children (Hess and Camara, 1979). Continued contact with the noncustodial parent appear to be beneficial to child and family adjustment so long as the noncustodial parent is not deviant or destructive. In situations where continued contact does have a positive effect on children, the ex-spouse relationships are characterized by an absence of mutual denigration and a high level of agreement on childrearing and discipline. Jacobson (1978) found that the loss of time with a noncustodial father was a strong predictor of maladjustment, although the quality of the relationship rather than the frequency of contact may be more important as a predictor of adjustment for some children.

There are specific types of parent-child relationships that appear to be related to the positive adjustment of children. Interactions between parents and children marked by high levels of communication and frequent expressions of warmth and caring, and infrequent expressions of negative, critical, or hostile affect, are associated with reduced stress in children and better social relations with peers. Additionally, the amount of time spent by parents in child-oriented activities is predictive of positive adjustment. When both parents remain involved in their child's social and school activity by meeting the child's friends and showing interest in their progress, children make a better adjustment to divorce. Although support from both parents appears to be optimal, a warm relationship with only one parent can help a child adjust to the stress of divorce (Hess and Camara, 1979).

Strategies that enable the child to maintain a positive relationship with each parent include the following: active and supportive involvement by both parents in childrearing; sharing information about children's accomplishments with the other parent or encouraging children to share their news (report cards, art projects, victories in a sports match); resisting impulses to denigrate the other parent whom the child may still love and respect; actively supporting the other parent in his or her role as father or mother; avoiding the temptation to use a child as a weapon in adult struggles; and attempting to reduce the amount of fighting that takes place when children are present (Camara, 1985; Hetherington, Cox, and Cox, 1982; McCall and Stocking, 1980).

PROVIDING A SECURE ENVIRONMENT

Problems in adjustment to divorce are least likely to occur when children are in predictable, secure environments, where parental discipline is both authoritative and consistent. In the first year after separation and divorce, the emotional distress experienced by family members often leads to diminished parental competence in the management of children's behavior. Parents communicate less well with the children, are less affectionate, less likely to monitor their children's disruptive and regressive behaviors, and are more likely to be erratic in establishing and maintaining limits.

The parents' feelings of reduced competence become exacerbated with the inevitable increase in household disorder, changes in routines, pressures of facing new jobs, reduced finances, and less time available for children. Parents' feelings of helplessness further contribute to the breakdown in child management and to the development of cycles of negative interactions between parents and children. In response, some parents have found it helpful to participate in programs designed to enhance their effectiveness by learning the use of contingent rewards and consistency in responding to children. These parents have found that instruction in techniques of managing children's behavior has resulted in fewer disciplinary problems, thus increasing parents' own self-esteem, reducing the anxiety felt by children, and breaking cycles of negative interactions. When parents set appropriate limits and use clear rules with explanation and discussion, the children are more likely to be well-adjusted. Permissive or authoritarian parent behaviors are correlated with poor adjustment in children (Hetherington, Cox, and Cox, 1982; Santrock and Warshak, 1979).

Parental functioning can also be restored through other means. Family counselors may help parents become more organized at home. Housekeeping support and dependable child care can give needed relief, assuming such help is available and affordable. Parent cooperative groups and neighborhood single-parent groups, where child care, transportation, and social support are shared among a group of parents faced with similar burdens, are alternatives for parents with limited resources and family supports.

REDEFINING ROLES

The changes accompanying the decision to divorce challenge the resources of even the healthiest of individuals and families, and require the flexibility and adaptability of family members in assuming new roles in the emergent family system. The ambiguity of post-divorce roles makes the transformation from a two-parent household to a two single-parent, two-household system difficult. Changes in living conditions, increased financial burdens, and the reduced availability of time available between parents and children represent environmental stressors that may negatively affect the redefinition of parental roles.

In addition to environmental stressors, parents and children may experience substantial role strain. This occurs when a single, custodial parent is required to assume the roles of the other parent in addition to her or his own role in the family. The single parent must be nurturer and disciplinarian. She or he may work outside the home as well as tend to the problems of daily household management. In some cases, children may need to take on some of the adult responsibilities (Weiss, 1979).

Noncustodial parents must attempt to redefine their roles as parents to their children, especially since the majority of noncustodial parents will have reduced contact with children following divorce. Role strain is inevitable in situations where cooperation between parents in childrearing issues is low and conflict is high. If one parent feels that the other is not an effective parent, he or she may actively work against the former spouse's child-management efforts. This situation may reinforce feelings of incompetence in each parent and may delay the emergence of satisfactory and appropriate parental and child roles in the family.

To assist family members in their struggle to identify new roles in the post-divorce family, Ahrons (1980) suggests the development of "binuclear" family systems where both parents play an active role in their children's lives. The process of role redefinition usually will include adult disengagement from spousal roles and the setting of rules to outline the ongoing coparental relationship. To the extent that parents are able to adjust and create a new family system, most children and adults will adapt to their changed family circumstances within a two-year period after divorce (Hetherington, Cox, and Cox, 1979; Wallerstein and Kelly, 1980). The coping of parents, particularly the noncustodial parent, is strongly associated with adjustment in children. The ease and success of the transition to a new family system will be in part dependent on the flexibility and adaptability of parents and the family's realistic acceptance of necessary changes.

SOCIAL SUPPORT

Social support received from friends, family, and community can be helpful to parents during the stressful years following divorce. While marital disruption can alter the types of personal support available to parents and children (Bohannen, 1971; Miller, 1971), relatives, particularly grandparents, may provide financial and emotional support to parents by caring for children and assisting them in handling problems of daily living and household management (Ahrons, 1981).

There is evidence to suggest that social support can protect adults and children against a variety of stressors and can promote recovery from crises (Caldwell and Bloom, 1982; Cobb, 1976). Such support is associated with less distress for members of divorced families (Coletta, 1979). Hetherington and her colleagues found that supports from parents, siblings, and close friends were related to the mother's effectiveness in responding to her children. The child's own sense of continuity and stability in the post-divorce family may depend on the continued availability of extended kin and extrafamilial supports (Kelly and Wallerstein, 1977). But what may constitute support in one situation may not in another, where parents or children feel trapped by a close social network or where the network is disapproving or unreliable (McLanahan, Wedemeyer, and Adelberg, 1981).

A variety of community services is available to families in most communities, but usually these are part of a more general mental health service that may not be designed for the specific needs of divorced parents and children. Even when divorce-specific resources are available, parents do not always use them (Camara, Baker, and Dayton, 1980). Welfare and community-based services are used selectively more often by lower-income than by moderate-income mothers (Coletta, 1979; Spicer and Hampe, 1975). Moderate-income parents may be more likely to discuss their concerns about children with relatives, friends, or in some cases family physicians. The increase in the use of health services by post-divorce families reported by Wertlieb and his colleagues (1984) suggests that parents may be more likely to seek consultation for physical, rather than psychological, symptoms evidenced during the post-separation period. Many parents report using these visits as an opportunity to discuss child-related psychological concerns (Wertlieb et al., 1984). Physicians are frequently unprepared to respond to such concerns and may refer parents to other sources of assistance.

Some parents have found it helpful to participate in short-term programs for newly separated parents or their children (Bloom, Hodges, and Caldwell, 1982; Weiss, 1975). Programs for parents may focus on adult issues related to the transition from married to single states or on the practical problems of daily living related to financial and household management. Some programs focus on child management and childrearing concerns.

Groups for children may focus on post-divorce family life, the adjustment to new schedules of contact with parents, and other difficulties. Such child groups can offer a safe place for children to discuss their feelings and to learn that their own experiences may not be unique (Kalter, Pickar, and Lesowitz, 1984). (For a comprehensive review of the types of programs and groups available to divorced families, see Baker et al., 1980.)

Thus far I have focused on factors related to the healthy adaptation to divorce and to the formation of a new family system. The role that each factor plays in promoting healthy adjustment of children is a function of the cognitive and social developmental level of the child. Whatever the circumstances of divorce and parental discord, it appears that children are upset by it in ways that vary with their age and developmental level. The competence of children at different developmental levels will limit the types of responses and coping strategies available to them. An examination of the developmentally related responses of children can help us to identify and preserve some of their "natural" coping processes.

The Child's Adjustment to Divorce

As emphasized earlier, there is great variability in children's vulnerability to marital disruption and interparental conflict. Empirical and clinical reports suggest that the establishment of close parent-child relationships, provision of secure environments, and the availability of personal and family supports can lead to more rapid and long-term adjustment of children. However, adaptations to post-divorce family life are profoundly influenced by the coping mechanisms available to children at each stage of development. The following discussion of children's responses to divorce draws from my own cross-sectional studies of children of different ages (Camara, 1979, 1985; Hess and Camara, 1979) and the results of two important longitudinal studies (Hetherington, Cox, and Cox, 1979; Wallerstein and Kelly, 1980.)

PRESCHOOL YEARS

Young children of preschool age, unable to understand the complexity of parental relationships, often are confused by parental discord and divorce. These children cannot see that others may have a perspective different from their own. They cannot comprehend how the loss of love or expression of anger between parents does not directly involve them. Egocentric in their understanding of their family and the world, young children may assume responsibility for parental fighting or divorce. They may blame themselves for having forgotten to put away their toys, believing their actions to be the cause of divorce. They may also believe that their actions and promises may bring parents back together again. It is not unusual for a young child to promise to be very good or to be more helpful so that a parent will return to the household.

Young children's symptoms of emotional stress take the form of nightmares, temper tantrums, bedwetting episodes, and expressions of unusual fears. They may engage in aggressive behaviors with their preschool peers or may withdraw from play with other children. Preschool boys, in particular, may display more pouting, clinging, and crying than do boys in families experiencing little or no family conflict. Somatic symptoms may develop as either conscious or unconscious attempts by children to attract their parents' attention or to distract them from angry interactions.

In response to the family tensions they experience, young children are likely to engage in elaborate fantasies about their parents' relationship. They see their parents as "good" and are unable to detect inconsistency or ambiguity in parental behaviors. These children may engage in play based on idealized concepts, pretending that parents still live together or that the children are still in close contact with a parent they may not have seen for several months. Many preschool children tend to buffer the stress of family discord by denying the presence of conflict.

Preschool children, dependent on the love and approval of their parents, may be unable to express their anger directly; instead they may engage in hostile negative fantasies within their play, scolding or punishing a doll that represents a parent or flushing a parent doll down the toilet. By engaging in these fantasies, young children seek temporary relief from the stresses they feel by expressing their anger and wishes within the safe context of play. These children may also focus on material losses experienced after divorce. Unable to identify the source of their feelings of loss and tension, they may describe such feelings of deprivation as not having so many toys now that Mommy and Daddy aren't together or not being able to go on a family trip. The displacement of feelings of loss may offer, at least temporarily, a concrete explanation for feelings of sadness and fears of abandonment in a situation they are unable to comprehend.

Although some have suggested that the effects of divorce may be more severe for younger children, there is no firm evidence to support this. Yet these children do have a more limited repertoire of coping processes, with fantasy, denial, self-blame, displacement, and somatic symptom development being the primary ways in which they respond to the stress in their lives. Counseling and support services need to be sensitive to these naturally occurring protective factors while reassuring children of their continued safety, protection, and parental love despite the family changes.

MIDDLE CHILDHOOD, EARLY YEARS

In the latency (early schoolyears) period of development, children are better able to identify the complexities of interpersonal relationships. In this period there is a distinct separation of one's own thoughts and those of others. Children can recognize the discrepancies between what they and their parents may be feeling. With an increased awareness comes an increased susceptibility to the stresses engendered by parental conflict. When divorce occurs during this stage of development, children are likely to experience intense feelings of sadness and, sometimes, despair. They may express anger toward one parent and are likely to use this anger as a defense against concern about the loss of a parent from their daily lives.

The growing ability to understand the feelings and perspectives of another allows them to be sympathetic and concerned for their parents. Latency-aged children are likely to identify with parents' views and thus become protective of parental feelings by concealing their own feelings from family and friends. They may become aligned with one parent or may feel conflicted in their loyalties to each parent.

Sometimes children of this age hold unrealistic perceptions of their involvement in either the initiation or the resolution of parental conflict. They are likely to attempt to referee fights. When parents stop speaking, children may try to organize an activity to force communication. They may make open bids to parents to stop fighting or arrange to have both parents present at special occasions in hopes of effecting a reconciliation. Avoidance of conflict and withdrawal from the tensions surrounding the divorce are strategies most often used by children of eight or nine years of age, once they have understood that they cannot solve their parents' problems or do anything to make them stop fighting. When I asked some seven- to nine-year-old children what they could do to make themselves feel better during parental arguments, they responded, "Run upstairs and block your ears," or "Read a book with the radio on so loud you can't hear them."

Although children of this age are better able to understand different perspectives, often they remain unaware of the silent tensions and subtle conflicts that exist between parents. Like preschool children, latency-aged children may be surprised by their parents' decision to divorce, especially when the conflicts are not overt or when fighting does not take place in front of the children. Their understanding of parental difficulties is limited to concrete signs of problems. When I showed children of this age a videotape of two arguing parents, they ascribed the reason for the fight to the specific content of words spoken and failed to detect the underlying meaning of the exchange.

MIDDLE CHILDHOOD, LATER YEARS

As children advance in age toward later stages of development, additional resources become available that may help to buffer the stresses of divorce. Children in the later elementary-school years may find alternative sources of gratification and support by participating with friends in extracurricular activities. Some children appear to block out the stress of parental conflict by immersing themselves in their schoolwork. Involvement in school or extracurricular activities offers a chance for these children to escape from family stresses and to obtain recognition from other adults or peers. Children in the later years of middle childhood may also use counseling services such as those offered by school guidance personnel. Many school programs offer counselor-led peer support groups for children whose parents are separating, divorcing, or remarrying.

Children of this age are better able to shift their reliance on parents to others outside the home. Frequently children in stressful home situations report spending large amounts of time in the homes of other families or with an adult friend or peer. The ability to remove themselves from parental conflict and to seek support from friends or other adults offers these children additional sources of strength in coping with family problems.

ADOLESCENCE

As children approach the adolescent years, they have an increased understanding of interpersonal conflict. With this comes different strengths and new tasks for those who are exposed to divorce. Adolescents no longer need to observe fighting in order to recognize the subtle conflicts that may exist between parents. On the other hand, their ability to recognize that others hold a different point of view may lead to greater self-consciousness, embarrassment, or fear of ridicule by peers.

The increased complexity of cognitive and social reasoning of adolescents allows them to evaluate authority figures more realistically than do younger children. The parent-child relationship is considered at this stage of development as both a reflection of and an influence on both parents' and children's personality and behavior. Questioning the role of parents as authority figures enables the adolescent to examine stressful situations more realistically and to understand the contribution that each person or condition makes to the overall situation. Adolescents, less reliant on parents to satisfy their needs, are more likely to be able to remove themselves from parental conflict. They may be able to forge separate relationships with each parent or to withdraw from the conflict. Their ability to examine simultaneously several aspects of a social situation allows them to separate the role that each family member may play in parental conflict.

Adolescents may react to the divorce with resentment and anger. For example, they may resent the added pressures and responsibilities placed on them at a time when they are beginning to develop a sense of belonging to their own peer group and are beginning to develop their relationships with opposite-sex peers. Visitation schedules with a noncustodial parent after divorce may be seen as interfering with their developing social lives. The adolescents' ability to hypothesize beyond real events may lead to a concern about their own future relationships, marriages, and expectations for parenthood. They are more likely than younger children to worry about their futures.

However, these older children do have a variety of supports and coping mechanisms available that can ease the process of adjusting to divorce. Adolescents whose parents are embroiled in bitter controversy or who are emotionally immobilized by the changes in their lives frequently assume the role of parent in the household, taking care of younger siblings and even the parents. The adults in the family depend upon these youngsters for support and advice. Although it has been suggested that such responsibility can lead to increased independence and maturity (Weiss, 1979), the responsibilities assumed by adolescents can often become burdensome. The reversal of child and parent roles can be developmentally disruptive and pose problems when adults in the household attempt to reassert their authority.

Many schools and communities now offer opportunities for adolescents to serve as peer leaders in support groups for troubled youth. Adolescents who have experienced parental conflict or divorce may become advisers to those in the midst of family problems and, as a result, gain a deeper understanding of their own family problems.

The ability of adolescents to interpret and restructure the meaning of past events enables them to recreate their family histories and propose solutions to problems based on their new retrospective understandings of their parents' conflicts. These adolescents may report that they are better off now that the parents have divorced. By recognizing each parent's weaknesses, the adolescent can adjust to divorce by developing separate relationships with each parent and a realistic acceptance of the divorce.

In sum, a variety of palliatives and problem-solving strategies in response to parental conflict and divorce become available to children at different points in their development. I have described the coping responses characteristic of children in each developmental period, although children at later developmental periods may use strategies from earlier stages. Children who are successful "adapters" will eventually discard any strategy that does not bring results. Children who are unable to discard maladaptive strategies or who are limited in the repertoire of adaptive mechanisms are more likely to experience difficulty. For example, an older elementary-school child who continues to use denial and fantasy in response to parental conflict will need extra help in order to achieve acceptance of the family situation. Programs and counseling services designed to help children in the midst of divorce and family change need to consider the coping processes of children at each developmental level, as well as the factors associated with healthy adjustment.

Implications for Future Policies

Divorce is a stressful process that brings with it other stresses, which may prove just as acute as the divorce itself to both children and parents. To the extent that those in the helping professions can provide a range of services that build on individual and family strengths and styles of coping, the adjustment to divorce may be eased.

Educational programs are needed for parents, children, and workers in the medical, mental health, legal, and teaching professions to alert them to potential difficulties, to help them understand the healthy responses each family member may have to divorce, and to identify signs of difficulty that may prevent or retard the development of a viable post-divorce family system. Unfortunately we know little about the effectiveness of different types of intervention programs designed to help parents, children, and families. We need systematic studies of the impact of educational, clinical, and self-help programs focused on individual and family coping.

We also need to identify and develop policies that will strengthen family life and contribute to the well-being of parents and children. Our future efforts must be directed toward the development of supports to mobilize family resources and build on individual and family strengths as parents and children accommodate to changes in their lives. Most important, we must be aware of policies and practices that weaken supports for families or increase risks for adults and children. Adversarial approaches to conflict resolution and support services that fail to consider the family as a whole need to be revised. There is no single clear solution to the problems encountered by children and parents in the midst of divorce. But increased collaboration and sharing of perspectives among professionals may lead to the development of comprehensive multidimensional plans to address the complex needs of the American family—in all its different forms.

JOHN M. LEVENTHAL and
BARBARA F. SABBETH

11 ✳

The Family and
Chronic Illness in Children

Raising a child with a chronic illness creates special problems and challenges for the family and its members. Parental expectations about the child's independence, the sick child's relation to healthy siblings, and the special services that may be required at school are a few of the many issues faced by the family in its effort to care for and live with a chronically ill child. Although for some families the struggle may be relatively easy and for others a constant uphill battle, for all families a chronic childhood illness is a major stress that can have a profound impact on both child and family. The focus of this chapter is on some of the special differences (Featherstone, 1980) faced by such families compared to families with healthy children and the challenges for clinicians as they care for such families.

Definition and Prevalence of Chronic Illness

As opposed to an acute illness in childhood, a chronic health condition has been defined as one lasting at least three months or requiring a period of hospitalization of at least one month's duration (Pless and Pinkerton, 1975). By such a definition it has been estimated that 10–15 percent of children have a chronic problem affecting their physical health and that 1–2 percent of all children have a severe chronic illness. Some of these children may be severely disabled and in constant pain, and some may die. When estimates of prevalence are based on the child's functioning, the 1981 National Health Interview Survey estimated that approximately two million children have some degree of limitation of normal activities (such as play); one million are limited in their ability to attend school; 95,000 cannot attend school; and 100,000 live in institutions (Newacheck et al., 1984).

Although a large number of children are affected by a chronic illness, the specific illnesses are usually rare. As shown in the list below (Gortmaker and Sappenfield, 1984), which presents prevalence estimates for 1980 of some of the most common childhood illnesses, asthma, sensory impairments, and mental retardation are the most common problems faced by children. Much less common are some of the well-publicized illnesses including congenital heart disease, myelomeningocele (spina bifida), sickle-cell disease, cystic fibrosis, and muscular dystrophy.

Clinicians are giving increasing amounts of time to the care of chronically ill children. This change in the pattern of care has

Disease	Prevalence (per 1000)
Asthma	
mild	28
severe	10
Visual impairment	
partial	30
total	0.6
Mental retardation	25
Hearing impairment	
partial	16
total	0.1
Congenital heart disease	7
Seizure disorder	3.5
Diabetes mellitus	1.8
Myelomeningocele	0.4
Sickle-cell anemia	0.3
Cystic fibrosis	0.2
Leukemia	0.1

come about for three main reasons. First, there has been a marked decrease in the morbidity and mortality in children from infectious illnesses because of improved living conditions, ready access to medical care, and the development and availability of potent antibiotics. Second, there has been an increase in the prevalence of chronic illnesses because of improvements in medical care and technology which have resulted in longer survival. For instance, the median age of survival for children with cystic fibrosis (the most common inherited, autosomal recessive disease in Caucasians, in the United States, with an estimated incidence of 1 in 2,000 births) was twenty years in 1981 compared to ten years in 1966 (Wood, 1984). Prolonged survival has resulted in new challenges: adolescents and young adults with cystic fibrosis have to make decisions about living away from home, going to college, or taking a job; children "cured" of leukemia have to live with concerns about possible relapse or the occurrence of new tumors at a rate higher than the general population. Third, technological advances in medical care have resulted in new forms of chronic illness. Children are now living with transplanted livers. Markedly premature infants are now surviving, some with handicapping conditions such as decreased visual acuity, mental retardation, or chronic lung problems. Technology, of course, is a double-edged sword. Advances in medical science have also resulted in a marked decrease in other chronic conditions, such as mental retardation, deafness, or heart disease from congenital rubella infection.

Caring for the Child

No matter how much a family protests that it treats a chronically ill child the same as a healthy one, there is always a difference in the care provided. Sometimes these differences are obvious, such as providing special transportation to school or excluding the child from certain activities of the family; other times they are subtle—restricting the distance an ill child is allowed to play away from home or tending to keep an ill child home from school with a minor illness. Raising a child with a chronic illness may affect at least four areas of care: (1) the parents' practical care of the child, (2) their feelings and attitudes toward the child, (3) how the family functions in its caring for the child, and (4) how the individual members of the family (including the child) manage their lives outside the home.

1. In terms of the practical aspects of care, families are faced with a myriad of tasks, many but not all of which can become routine while others can become a constant source of friction and difficulty. Take, for example, the care of a child with diabetes mellitus. Daily care requires one to two injections of insulin per day, checking glucose levels in the urine or blood four times a day, a special diet, and regular exercise. Parents (and eventually the children themselves) have to make appropriate adjustments in the dosage of insulin and be vigilant of the signs of hypo- or hyperglycemia. Extra expenses related to daily care would include insulin, syringes, and materials and equipment for testing. The approximate 1985 cost to provide this care was $1,000 a year (Davis, 1985). Although many families manage these special demands, in other families diets are not followed or testing is done irregularly, resulting in poor diabetic control. For some families a second job may be necessary to meet the additional expenses.

Daily care of children with other illnesses may be still more complicated and time-consuming. The child may require assistance in dressing, eating, or toileting; in others, expert care such as that provided by nursing or physical therapy may be necessary. Such expert care will become increasingly common as more children with chronic illnesses receive intensive medical care at home (Association, 1984).

The child's illness may require frequent visits to pediatric specialists and/or frequent hospitalizations. While medical insurance might cover some or most of the medical costs, it does not cover the costs of traveling to the medical center, the babysitters to watch the children at home, staying in the hospital with the sick child, or time lost from work. An illness may restrict the family's social activities outside the home and may affect job mobility or moves because of the necessity to stay near centers of medical care.

2. Caring for an ill child affects parental attitudes and feelings toward the child. Whether a child is born with a congenital anomaly or becomes ill later in life, parents experience a similar grieving process. This process involves mourning the loss of the normal, healthy child—either the child that was hoped for or the child that the family had known as normal until the diagnosis (Solnit and

Stark, 1961). The task may be psychologically more difficult than grieving a death in the family because parents have to give up their view of their child as normal and, at the same time, accept the child with his or her chronic condition. Certainly how the parents work their way through this process will affect how they come to terms with their child's problems. Even parents who have adjusted well will have recurrent episodes of sadness, especially at important times (as when the child is hospitalized). Olshansky (1962) has called the process one of chronic grief.

Contradictory feelings may sometimes exist at the same time. Parents may want to protect the helpless sick child but still feel revulsion at the child's abnormality. Parents may love the child but also feel guilty or angry at their child or spouse for "causing" the problem (MacKeith, 1973). It would be an error to underestimate the parents' feelings of embarrassment with family or friends because the child is different.

3. Several important tasks are involved in the care of the chronically ill child in a family. First and foremost is the integration of this child into family life. How to include this child in the family's special activities or trips requires ingenuity and sometimes special expenses. Preparing one kind of food for the ill child and another for the rest of the family may make the child feel isolated and like an outsider. Secrets about the illness may isolate the child. Honest and age-appropriate communication between the parents, between the parents and the ill child, and among the siblings and sick child and parents is a crucial yet difficult task (Leventhal et al., 1984). Special challenges in communication among family members might arise when a school-age child with a chronic illness sees a televised appeal to help raise money for his own illness and the appeal indicates that the money will help prevent early deaths or prevent crippling paralysis. How should parents handle this problem?

A chronic illness may make it more difficult to accomplish other tasks such as including the siblings, maintaining the marriage, and providing time for the individual growth of family members (Leventhal, 1984). Caring for a sick child may require so much time and physical and emotional energy that these other tasks may be ignored or given less emphasis.

4. Caring for a chronically ill child also involves important tasks outside the home. For a child, the major activities outside the home

are at school and with friends. These activities may be particularly difficult for the child with a chronic illness who may be sheltered at home, may have difficulty with separations, and may be embarrassed about his defect and have problems forming friendships (Weitzman, 1984). Going to school and interacting with peers will affect parents as well. Parents have to allow the child appropriate independence—but it might be difficult if not impossible for the parents of a child with a seizure disorder to let the child out of their sight to play down the street with friends. Whereas sending a child to school is often straightforward and uncomplicated, for families with a sick child there may be additional burdens, including paperwork, meetings, or class visits to ensure that the child is in the right classroom setting. It may be very difficult for parents who have spent so much time providing expert care and nurturance to their child to rely on the seemingly superficial judgments of others. Pitched battles over placement or expectations may ensue.

Throughout the parents' and child's contacts with the outside world, there is the special stress of being different. Gliedman and Roth (1980) call it the "shameful differentness." What results is the stigmatization that occurs when someone observes the physical condition and assumes mental and social deviance. How the family manages this issue is vital to how the child and the other members of the family function outside the home.

Care and Adjustment

Factors that influence how a family is able to care for a child and adjust to the child's illness are outlined schematically in the accompanying figures. The first, which presents a static model, indicates that the child's illness does not exist in a vacuum. Some of the major characteristics for each of the levels in the figure are listed

ECOLOGY OF PARENTING

below. To indicate the importance of these characteristics, consider these examples. The first example concerns the parents' own background. Parents who have had experience with a chronic illness in childhood, either as patients or as family members, may have particular expectations for their own ill children. Such parents may be highly empathic or unusually tough. One diabetic father we interviewed in a study of families with a diabetic child felt that, since he made it to adulthood without special attention, his son should be able to do the same. The second example highlights the importance of characteristics of the social setting and cultural context. The availability of both nonhealth and health-related services

Child
    age and sex
    intelligence
    personality attributes
    ability to form relations

Parents
  As individuals
    own nurturing
    previous experience with stress
    importance of religion
    medical and psychiatric problems
    "success" in own life
  As parents
    relations with child
    meaning of illness to parents

Family
    structure
    marital relation
    other relations
    financial resources
    support systems

Social setting and cultural context
    poverty
    availability of health services
    availability of other services
    attitudes toward handicap

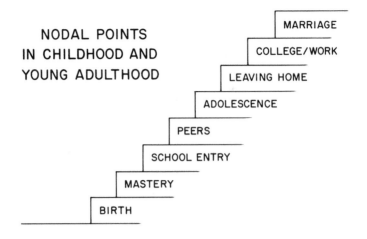

NODAL POINTS
IN CHILDHOOD AND
YOUNG ADULTHOOD

MARRIAGE

COLLEGE/WORK

LEAVING HOME

ADOLESCENCE

PEERS

SCHOOL ENTRY

MASTERY

BIRTH

can have a dramatic effect on the child and family. Such services might include a special preschool program for handicapped children, special transportation, special services (such as physical therapy) in the school, a home care program, or coordinated medical care at a large tertiary medical center.

Our second figure shows a dynamic model of a child's and young adult's development. The way a family functions in relation to the child and the illness depends in part on the child's development at the onset of the illness and the subsequent interactions of the illness and these developmental stages. For instance, in a recent study of parents of children with diabetes or cystic fibrosis, we found that the mothers' communication with their children about the illness was similar for both diseases but that fathers communicated more effectively to the child with diabetes than to the child with cystic fibrosis (Leventhal et al., 1984). One possible explanation for this difference in communication is the timing of the onset of the disease. Since children with cystic fibrosis are usually symptomatic during the first year of life, perhaps fathers withdraw from these ill infants and are never able to form a good relationship with their children. In contrast, children with diabetes are older at the age of onset and fathers have had an opportunity to establish a relationship before the illness strikes.

Together, the models outlined in the figures provide a framework for the clinician. The first is a reminder of those variables that influence the child and family at any one time; the second, that the child's illness presents different hurdles to the child and family over the course of the child's lifetime.

One additional set of characteristics, those related to illness, can have an impact on the functioning of child and family:

— age of onset
— course of the illness (static vs. relapsing)
— prognosis
— visibility
— extent of pain
— limitations of mobility
— cognitive functioning involved
— sensory functioning involved
— genetic disease
— extent of care

For example, it may be much easier for a child to develop relations with peers if the illness is relatively invisible (say diabetes) compared to an illness that is visible or disfiguring (spina bifida) The visibility of an illness is complicated and depends on the eye of the beholder. A child with epilepsy has an illness that is usually invisible, but one grand mal seizure will make it quite apparent to classmates. In contrast, a child with a chest scar from open heart surgery may have an invisible illness in that his peers cannot see the surgical scar, but the child himself may feel quite different and believe that people can see the scar and the differentness even through a shirt and sweater.

Adjustment of Families

How well do children with a chronic illness and their families function? Implicit in this question is the notion that the additional stress caused by the illness results in malfunctioning. Although some investigators have found no differences between the functioning of families with a chronic illness and families without an illness, in general investigators have found that families facing a chronic illness have more psychosocial problems (the child has a school problem or the parent is depressed) than families without this additional stress. Many families also have been studied who manage and cope well.

Because human behaviors and feelings are being assessed, the answer to the question is of course a complicated one and depends in part on the following issues:

1. What is meant by "adjustment"? The term can refer to several areas of functioning in the child and/or family. For instance, when investigating a child's adjustment to an illness, one could assess the child's moods and feelings (depression or self-esteem), the child's behavior at home, or the child's behavior at school and with friends. Often investigators will assess one or two areas of functioning and conclude that, because the child and/or family is doing well in those areas, the family is psychologically well adjusted. Such conclusions obviously can be hazardous.

2. What is meant by "good" adjustment? When describing adjustment, clinicians and researchers often refer to individuals or families as well adjusted or poorly adjusted. Many measures of adjustment provide a cutoff score, below which a subject is considered to be poorly adjusted (say a parent who scores in the depressed region on a depression inventory or a child whose behavior falls in the problem region on a behavioral inventory). The issue is more complicated, however. Take young adults with cystic fibrosis. Many continue to live with their families of origin; some have tried living at college but have returned home. They are not preparing themselves for independence in the ways expected of others their age. Their parents are more involved in their lives than expected under more ordinary circumstances. Are these families poorly adjusted or well adjusted given the prognosis of the ill child?

3. What measures are used to assess adjustment? Pless and Pinkerton (1975) have summarized the various approaches to assessing the adjustment of a chronically ill child. Different results can be obtained depending on how one assesses a particular area of functioning. For instance, when assessing depression in children, parents' and childrens' reports provide different information (Weissman et al., 1980; Moretti et al., 1985).

4. Who is serving as a comparison group? Many of the earlier studies were conducted without suitable control groups so that it was difficult to tell if the rate of maladjustment in chronically ill children and their families was higher than in families without a chronic illness. More recently, comparison groups with healthy

children have been employed. Some have suggested that it is inappropriate to use behaviors of nondisabled children in normative studies, but without such comparisons it would be impossible to assess the extent of the problems and to determine where clinicians should focus their efforts.

5. Who in the family is being assessed? A chronic disease can have a different impact on each member of the family. The child with the illness may be doing reasonably well while the sibling is having marked difficulties.

6. When during the course of the illness is the evaluation being conducted? A recent article in the *New England Journal of Medicine* describes the outcome of children with spina bifida who were followed from birth to school age (McLaughlin et al., 1985). Outcomes included IQ scores, the ability to ambulate, and whether the child was living at home. Gross's editorial in the same issue provides a reminder that the outcomes as described are only part of the story— "the rest of the story," as the editorial was titled, is of greater importance. How will these children function as young adults and how will their families function? As adults, how many will live independently of their families, have adequate mobility, have a job, and be able to form intimate relationships?

With these caveats in mind, we will briefly review what is known about the adjustment of child and family to a chronic illness. More extensive reviews are available in the literature (Pless and Pinkerton, 1975; Haggerty, 1984; Blacher, 1984).

Adjustment of the Child

Children with a chronic illness, as might be expected, have more behavioral and social problems. Pless and Roghmann (1971) reviewed the findings from three large epidemiological studies that compared rates of psychosocial problems in chronically ill and healthy children. The populations for the studies were: the total population of nine- to eleven-year-old children on the Isle of Wight, England; the National Survey of Health and Development, which followed a representative sample of children born in the United Kingdom in 1946 through their fifteenth birthday; and the Rochester Child Health Survey, which consisted of a 1 percent probability sample of children living in Monroe County, New York. In each population, the chronically ill children had more psychosocial problems, although the measures of adjustment were often quite different. For example, in the Isle of Wight study, 17 percent of chronically ill children had a psychiatric disorder (based on a psychiatrist's assessment) compared to 7 percent in the healthy children. Questionnaires completed by parents and teachers about the child's behaviors showed similar rates of deviant scores. In the National Survey, 25 percent of chronically ill children versus 17 percent of controls had at least two abnormal behavioral symptoms as reported by parents. In the Rochester survey, 30 percent of chronically ill children aged eleven through fifteen had at least two abnormal behavioral symptoms compared to 13 percent of the controls. Children with chronic illnesses also had more problems with school performance and were more often truant, considered troublesome in school, and were socially isolated.

Studies of smaller populations and with specific illnesses have in general confirmed these results. For instance, Hoare (1984) showed that children with epilepsy (both those recently diagnosed and those with chronic epilepsy) had markedly elevated rates of psychiatric disturbances on parent and teacher rating scales (approximately 45 percent) compared to children with diabetes (17 percent) and healthy controls (10 percent). In contrast, Drotar (1981) claimed that children with cystic fibrosis did not have excessive rates of psychosocial disturbances. In fact, he found that 19 percent of these children were reported by their mothers to have behavioral disturbances; this rate was almost four times the rate (5 percent) in the healthy comparison group.

We believe that the evidence is convincing: children with chronic illness do have more psychosocial problems; the rates in chronically ill children may be two to three times higher than in healthy children. It is also clear that most children with chronic illness do not have *serious* psychosocial problems. Why the majority of these children do well and how they go about living with their illness is an area for further exploration.

Children with chronic illness also miss more school than healthy children. Fowler (1985) reviewed school records of 270 children with chronic illnesses followed at eleven pediatric specialty clinics in Chapel Hill, North Carolina. On average, these children missed sixteen days of school (range 0 to 164) compared with the state norm of less than seven days. According to parents, children missed school because of minor illnesses, the chronic health condition itself, or clinic visits. Children with hemophilia, arthritis, or asthma were most often absent because of the illness itself. The findings of this and other studies on chronic illness and school absenteeism are not unexpected. When children miss school, they often fall behind in their work and sometimes fail to get promoted. Thus school failure may become an additional burden for children with chronic illness.

Some investigators have wondered whether the type of illness affects the likelihood of a child's developing a psychosocial problem. Pless and his colleagues have attempted to classify illnesses into three groups according to the social aspect of the disability: those with a sensory handicap (say hearing impairment), those with a visible (cosmetic) defect compromising the child's appearance (cleft lip), and those that interfere with physical functioning but are not visible (congenital heart disease) (Pless, 1983; Heller et al., 1985). Pless hypothesized that children with a sensory deficit would have the highest rates of psychosocial maladjustment, and the results of several studies support this hypothesis.

Similar questions have been raised with regard to the severity of an illness. Unfortunately, the concept of biologic severity is not always clear-cut and may be associated with compliance. For instance, a child with frequent asthmatic attacks may have a severe degree of asthma or may not be taking the prescribed medications to prevent attacks. When severity is considered, clinicians intuitively believe that children with more severe disease in terms of biological handicaps are more likely to have psychosocial problems. Some have raised the intriguing possibility that children with mild disease may also have marked psychosocial problems. For example, McAnarney and her colleagues (1974) found that 42 percent of children with mild disability from juvenile rheumatoid arthritis were considered maladjusted, compared to 38 percent of those whose disability was severe. To explain this finding the authors and others have suggested that children who are at the border or margin between well and sick may have difficulty adjusting to this role.

One final area of concern is the long-term impact of chronic illness. As more children with chronic illness are "cured" and more live into adulthood with their disabilities, what will their lives be like as adults? Systematic research to answer this question is just beginning. For example, one large follow-up study conducted by Koocher and O'Malley (1981) examined 121 survivors of childhood cancer. These young adults were subject to medical risks, such as the increased rate of secondary tumors, and to the long-term effects of treatment, such as delayed puberty, sterility, or scars and amputations from surgery. In terms of mental health, many had no impairment, but a quarter had mild psychological symptoms, 10 percent had moderate symptoms, and 11 percent had severe symptoms. As medical treatments improve and more psychosocial services are provided for the children and their families, the medical and psychological health of survivors is likely to improve as well.

Adjustment of the Family

Most studies of the adjustment of families to chronic childhood illness have focused on individuals rather than the family system. Mothers of chronically ill children have been reported to have a high occurrence of depression (Allan et al., 1974; Walker, et al., 1971), which is not too surprising given the tremendous difficulties and loneliness they can experience in caring for the child. In a well-controlled study, Breslau (1985) showed that mothers of chronically ill children had significantly higher scores on scales of depression-anxiety and maternal distress compared to mothers of healthy children. The scores were not affected by the type of disability. Mothers also have been reported to feel physically tired, guilty, and isolated, and to worry about their child's future.

Less is known about how fathers respond to a child's illness, but their range of responses should be similar to those of mothers. Fathers may have more difficulty participating in the child's daily care and are more likely to withdraw from the child (Cummings, 1976; Sabbeth et al., 1984). Sometimes work or philanthropic activities may become a safety zone away from the family and the pain. Other fathers work shorter hours to spend more time with their families and give up job advancements so they do not have to relocate.

Siblings, too, feel the effects of a chronically ill child in the home.

They may assume extra responsibilities and may be neglected by parents. Siblings may resent the extra attention given to the sick child. They may be angry toward the parents and competitive with the sick child; they also may be ashamed of the sick child and the situation created in the family. Several systematic studies have been conducted about the adjustment of siblings compared to those without an illness in the family. Although a few investigators have found that siblings were more poorly adjusted than the controls (Tew and Laurence, 1973; Vance et al., 1980), others have found no differences (Breslau et al., 1981; Lavigne and Ryan, 1979). One possible explanation for the failure to find differences is that maladjustment is usually assessed by parental reports of the siblings' behavior; if parents are concentrating their attentions on the sick child, they might underestimate and underreport the problematic behaviors of the healthy siblings. Future studies should obtain information from parents as well as from the healthy siblings themselves.

The effects of the chronic illness on the parents' marriage have been explored in many studies, but often in a superficial manner. In a recent review of thirty-four published papers that investigated the effects of chronic illness on marital adjustment, we found that divorce rates in families with a chronic illness were not substantially higher than in control families (Sabbeth and Leventhal, 1984). In contrast, there was an increased amount of marital distress, indicating that the illness made it difficult for parents to maintain the quality of their marriage. Much less is known about other areas of marital adjustment, such as communication between spouses, decision making, and role flexibility.

Few investigators have examined other relations in the family or the family system. We recently investigated how parents communicate with their sick child about the illness (Leventhal et al., 1984). Parents of children with diabetes or cystic fibrosis have minimal communication with their children about the illness. Such parents seem to maintain secrecy in the family, perhaps to protect themselves and the children from painful information. It seemed to us that protection was often valued above honesty.

Other investigators have taken a systems view of families. Lewis and Khaw (1982) studied family functioning in three groups of children: cystic fibrosis, asthma, and healthy controls. They showed that family functioning, when measured on the dimensions of cohesion and adaptability (Olson et al., 1979), was similar in all three groups and that family functioning was a better predictor of child adjustment than was the presence of illness. In studies of seriously ill children with diabetes and asthma who were extremely difficult to manage, Minuchin and his colleagues have described "psychosomatic families" (Liebman et al., 1974). Such families are characterized by enmeshment, overprotectiveness, rigidity, and lack of conflict resolution. The sick child plays an important role in the family's avoidance of conflict, and the child's symptoms do not improve until the family organization has been changed.

In summary, although much has been learned about the psychosocial impact of chronic illness on families, there are still important gaps in our knowledge. Special attention should be paid to understanding the effects on fathers and how to include fathers in the clinical care. Also we know little about the strengths in families and why certain families adjust well.

Financial Impact

The financial burden on a family with a chronically ill child can be staggering. Medical expenses include the cost of hospitalizations, physicians' services, diagnostic tests, medications, self-care procedures, and special services such as social services, home nursing, or respite care. Nonmedical expenses include the costs of transportation, extra telephone calls, time lost from work, special diets, and special costs such as structural modifications in the home. Although each family with a chronic illness does not incur all of these costs, it is clear that costs are concentrated in a small proportion of families. Fr example, only 5.4 percent of children, many of whom were chronically ill, were hospitalized at least once in 1978 (Perrin and Ireys, 1984). Compared to the average yearly expense of $286 for health care of children in 1978, the cost for an average hospitalization was $1,920. When the health resources utilized by children are examined, 2–3 percent of children use 40% of the resources.

To get a better idea of the costs related to specific illnesses, Perrin and Ireys (1984) present figures on two diseases. The average cost for the first weeks of life for an infant born with spina bifida is

$6,500; the average total cost in 1980 for the first two years of life was $70,000. For hemophilia, the average yearly costs of medical care for children and adults living in Tennessee in 1978 was $8,071 (range $0 to $56,000).

Many of the costs of medical care are covered by private medical insurances, Medicaid, or Crippled Children's Services. Still families must pay a substantial amount of medical costs and most nonmedical costs. For example, out-of-pocket expenses were 12 percent of family income for families with spina bifida (Perrin and Ireys, 1984). When lost income and nonmedical costs were included, out-of-pocket expenses rose to 25 percent. Such costs, obviously, can impose a tremendous financial burden on families.

Medical and Psychosocial Care

Providing clinical care can be a true challenge. On the one hand, clinicians try to offer the children and their families medical care that includes the most up-to-date approaches to prevention, detection, and cure. But, as indicated throughout this chapter, biomedical care alone is not enough. To help families overcome the impact of the illness, psychosocial care also is necessary, including psychosocial services, education, and rehabilitation. The goals of such care are twofold: first, to prevent serious sequelae such as school failure or low self-esteem and, second, to detect problems early so that appropriate interventions can be provided. Psychosocial services that can be helpful to families include parent education, genetic counseling, homemaker services, respite care, mental health counseling, parent groups, and lay counselors (Pless and Satterwhite, 1972). In addition, children may need special services in school, such as speech and language therapy, transportation, and counseling. With the enactment of Federal Law 94-142 in 1978, such services, if necessary, must be provided to handicapped children (Walker, 1984).

A major clinical and policy question is how best to provide the necessary care in an efficient and coordinated fashion. Many children now receive the care for their chronic illness at tertiary medical centers where a team often provides the care: the pediatric specialists provide the leadership and medical expertise while the nurse-practitioner and social worker provide the coordination and psychosocial services. In other cases, the child's pediatrician provides most of the care and coordination, and the pediatric specialist is used only as a consultant for medical problems. In still other cases, particularly those in which children have multiple handicaps, care is often not coordinated; families make multiple trips to the hospital, see different specialists, and no psychosocial care is provided.

Other models of care have tried to improve the coordination and psychosocial components of care. Stein and Jessop (1984) have evaluated a home care program for children with chronic illnesses living in the Bronx. Care is provided by a nurse-practitioner, generalist pediatrician, and social worker both in the home and in the clinic. The results of a clinical trial demonstrated that this program was successful in improving the family's satisfaction with care and the child's psychological adjustment, and in decreasing the mother's psychiatric symptoms. A different approach to providing necessary services is the Chronic Health Impaired Program (CHIP), which was developed in Baltimore in the mid-1970s (Case and Mathews, 1983). Since children with chronic illnesses often miss school, this program was designed to increase school attendance, decrease the rate of nonpromotion, and maintain academic achievement. By providing special CHIP teachers to secure the homework of the sick child who missed school and to instruct them in the home or hospital, the program was able to decrease the rate of nonpromotions from 12.0 percent to 2.9 percent. Special programs also have been developed to provide coordinated regional care (Pierce and Freedman, 1983).

Regardless of how care is provided, it is clear that children with a chronic illness and their families often need many types of services. The goals of these services are the same: to minimize both the biological deficit and the psychosocial consequences of that deficit. If services are provided in a successful way, then the child with a handicap will not become a handicapped child living in a handicapped family and will not grow up to become a handicapped adult.

12 ✳

Teenage Pregnancy

Pregnancy causes significant stress under any circumstances. Even when the pregnancy is intended, the male and female partner are married, and the woman is in the traditional childbearing years, pregnancy and the first few years with a child are difficult and require a range of supports if major problems are to be avoided.

These stresses and the range of supports needed are multiplied when pregnancy occurs in a woman who is still of school age. In this situation, the mother's age, marital status, and attitudes toward pregnancy and childbearing are frequently less than optimal. For example, women under the age of twenty are at higher risk for pregnancy complications than are older women, and their children are more likely to be of low birth weight. In addition, school-age mothers are frequently unmarried and their pregnancies, regardless of marital status at delivery, are less likely to be intended. Not surprisingly, many teenage pregnancies end in abortions.

Fortunately, despite references to an epidemic, the number of teenage births is on the decline. The rise in the number of births to females under the age of eighteen during the early 1970s reflected not only the increase in teenage sexual activity that began in the previous decade, but also the larger number of teenage women. The children of the postwar baby boom entered their teenage years in the 1960s and 1970s and thus, even if the amount of sexual activity had remained low and stable, the number of teenage pregnancies would have increased. The combination of more individuals at risk and a rise in sexual activity among teenagers has resulted in many years when there were over a million teenage pregnancies (although the availability of abortion reduced the number of births). Some studies have also reported greater use of family-planning methods among teenagers (Zelnik and Kantner, 1980; Forest, Hermalin, and Henshaw, 1981).

Of particular concern to those interested in family dynamics is the number of teenage births that are out of wedlock and, therefore, place significant burdens on the young mother, her family, and the newborn. In 1978 it was estimated that for every 100 teenage pregnancies, 13 ended in miscarriages, 38 in induced abortions, 27 in births within marriage, whether premaritally or postmaritally conceived, and 22 in births outside marriage (Alan Guttmacher Institute, 1981). Very few teenagers in this last group relinquish their infants for adoption: less than 10 percent of white teenagers and an even smaller percentage of black teenagers. Thus, over the last few years, approximately a quarter of a million teenagers a year have joined the ranks of those who face the stresses of raising an infant without the support of a husband.

The Stresses

Although some pregnant teenagers share quarters with friends, male or female, and some live in institutions for the retarded, disturbed, or delinquent, most live at home with one or both parents. Almost invariably, the news of a pregnancy in this situation is cause for disappointment and dismay. Even in social groups where unmarried adolescent pregnancy is common or when the grandmother-to-be was herself an unmarried teenage mother, the parents usually hoped that their children's experiences would be different. In groups where such a pregnancy is uncommon, the shock is even greater.

These psychological stresses are soon followed by financial and physical ones. During the pregnancy, medical care and the need for more food and new clothes for the pregnant woman may cause economic problems, partially offset in some households by welfare payments. After the baby is born, financial burdens usually increase; and unless the family has, or can obtain, adequate living accommodations, some loss of space and privacy is almost inevitable.

In addition, many family members may be called upon to share responsibility for the baby, especially if the teenager is very young or for other reasons perceived as lacking the ability to care adequately for the child. If the teenager chooses to return to school or to work after the baby is born, large demands for child-care assistance may be placed on grandmother and siblings.

But it is the young mother herself who usually experiences the greatest stress. With the tasks of adolescence not yet completed, she must assume the burdens of adulthood. The normal problems involved in disengaging from one's family in order to become an independent adult are compounded by the need for assistance, which causes a continuation of dependence. Issues of continuing her relationship with the baby's father and of returning to school may also place stress on the adolescent.

These stresses may be increased by conflicts between the young mother and other family members. Pre-pregnancy areas of disagreement may be heightened: for example, parent-child quarrels about responsibility for household duties, schoolwork, or how often or how late the teenager should stay out. And new areas of conflict may emerge. Most critical perhaps are disagreements about the care of the infant. Grandmother and mother may argue about feeding, clothing, care of minor ailments, and a variety of other issues. Another problem area may be the role of the young father. Should he be encouraged to see the new mother and their child and treated as one of the family, or should he be kept away as punishment or to prevent another pregnancy?

Positive Aspects

Some young mothers report that the pregnancy and newborn period has positive aspects as well. The young mother's status in the family often improves. She is treated with additional respect, more like an adult. Furstenberg (1981) quoted one of the black teenage mothers in his study as saying that she was treated less like a girl and more like a woman. Schwab (1983) found similar benefits for the young mothers in her poor, rural, white New Hampshire sample. The title of her thesis, "Some One to Always Be There," suggests one positive aspect of early childrearing in a physically and often emotionally impoverished area. She mentions several others: "The strategy of early entrance into motherhood is rational adaptive because it brings short-term benefits, such as access to material resources, achievement of adult status, independence from parents, and power in relationships with men."

Many grandmothers also seem to enjoy the new baby, at least in the first few months. Furstenberg found that it had a "rejuvenating" effect on some. One adolescent mother reported that her mother felt younger since the baby's birth. The grandmother herself said she was "happier inside . . . not as nervous." An article in *MS* magazine (Leishman, 1980) featured a white teenager, her baby, and her mother, and quoted the mother as saying: "Well, she wanted to keep the baby—none of us believes in abortion— and she didn't want to get married which was okay with us. After all, fifteen is kind of young to marry and we wanted her to finish high school and go to college. Anyway, I've had ten kids, so as long as I can remember there's always been a baby in the house, and this one is our pride and joy."

A few families report a general improvement in relations following the birth of the child. Husbands (now grandfathers) as well as siblings (now aunts and uncles) may become more responsible because of the demands placed on them by the baby. Recent studies have suggested that the father of the new baby, even if he is not married to the young mother, may attempt to assist her emotionally and financially (Barret and Robinson, 1982; Brown, 1983, Hendricks and Montgomery, 1983). The strength and duration of these activities, however, has been questioned (Lorenzi, Klerman, and Jekel, 1977).

Levy and Grinker (1982) documented many types of stress, as well as several sources of support, in their ethnographic study of pregnant and parenting teenagers who were participating in Project Redirection, a multiservice program for such youngsters. In their summary, they supported many of the statements made earlier:

> The teens turned increasingly to their mothers for support during pregnancy and after delivery. Although in many cases they initially disapproved of the pregnancy, the mothers were responsive to their daughters' needs, often providing child care and other kinds of financial and emotional support.

The closeness of the mother/daughter relationship by no means meant that it was free of tension. The girls in this sample were caught in an adolescent dilemma common to most teenagers in this society: confusion about whether they were children or adults, whether they sought freedom or nurturance. Their new status as mothers and mothers-to-be served to exacerbate the conflict, raising such issues as whether it was they or their mothers who were primarily responsible for care of the baby, or whether their mothers had the right to set the rules about what care should be given. Nevertheless, these conflicts were rarely so strong that they severed connections between mothers and daughters.

Generally, the teens were far less involved with their fathers than their mothers. Many fathers were wholly absent from the household or present only intermittently. Many had been involved in crime or were financially dependent. Even in intact two-parent households, they seldom offered a positive male image to the teens.

The families of the teens rarely encouraged them to marry the fathers of their babies. This held true for all ethnic groups, even the more traditional Mexican-American families. Every teen and all but one of the families decisively rejected the option of adoption. Such reactions are consistent with recent observations that there is increased acceptance of single motherhood in contemporary society.

Although a number of the relationships were stormy, many of the teens continued to be involved with the fathers of their babies during the period of this study. Few fathers denied their paternity. Many provided support, either financial or emotional or both, to the mother and her baby.

None of the teens, however, chose to marry the father of the baby during this study period. Even among those who began the pregnancy with the intention of marrying the father, all seemed to conclude that marriage to this particular young man at this particular point in their lives would not solve their needs for long-term emotional and financial support.

Negative Reactions

Obviously not all families are supportive—in fact, the teenagers just described may have been able to participate in Project Redirection only because their families were supportive. Some teenagers have mothers who say, "You made your bed and now you must lie in it," and refuse to give help and support. Other teen-agers' fathers or mothers cannot deal with the shame they perceive to be associated with illegitimacy and try to separate themselves from the erring adolescent. Often siblings tease or make fun of the pregnant adolescent or share the sense of shame and seek to isolate themselves from her. Male partners' reactions may vary from support to flight, to insistence on abortion, to violence.

Most pregnant adolescents, however, probably underestimate their parents' capacity to deal with an unintended pregnancy. The teenager's cry, "I can't go home—my parents will kill me," is usually an exaggeration. After the initial shock many families accept the situation and adapt to it. A counselor for Planned Parenthood (Taves, 1983) described her role-playing approach to this situation as follows:

> If the girl says, "She'd kill me," or "They'd kill me," I'll say, "It sounds like they'd be upset—how would they react?" Girl: "My mom would say, 'How could you do this to me?' " Me: "How long would that last?" Girl: "About five minutes." Me: "What would you be doing during that?" Girl: "Crying and just waiting for it to be over." Me: "Then what?" Girl: "She probably put her arms around me and we'd cry together." It helps her decide whether the problem is telling the family or how they'd react.

But some fathers, brothers, and boyfriends become abusive, so service providers must make it clear to pregnant and parenting adolescents that such actions should not be tolerated as normal, transient, or deserved. The adolescent should be encouraged to contact the provider should violence be threatened or actually occur. Advice and temporary shelter should be available to deal with this problem. And maternity homes, foster-care placements, and alternative living arrangements should also be provided by the community for the youngster whose family forces her out as a result of anger or shame over the pregnancy.

The reasons why some families are supportive during the crisis of adolescent parenting and pregnancy, and others are not, are still unknown. Probably families from social and ethnic back-grounds in which pregnancy at young ages is common tolerate the situation better. Also families that live in areas with high rates of teenage pregnancies may be more accepting. These would include both inner-city ghettos and enclaves of rural poverty. Such families share a sense of despair about the future. If a family does not believe that education, vocational training, or other future-oriented activity will make a difference to its daughter's eventual lifestyle, then it may be more accepting of the pregnancy. It is among those families who had planned for their daughters' futures that stress may be highest and that support may be withheld. Another characteristic that may separate supportve and unsupportive families is a family's fundamentalist religious beliefs. If pemarital sexual activity is perceived as sinful, it may be difficult to support the errant family member.

The impact of support and conflict on a small sample of pregnant adolescents was studied by Barrera (1981). He found that the size of the conflicted network—individuals who provided at least one support function but who were also sources of interpersonal conflict—was positively correlated with symptoms of maladjustment, including anxiety. But the association between stressful life events and symptoms was less for those adolescents with larger total and unconflicted networks.

Support Services

Research is needed to determine the factors that make some families supportive and others rejecting. The findings of such studies may enable service providers to prevent some of the psychological and occasionally physical trauma that pregnant and parenting teenagers sometimes endure. Meanwhile, however, social agencies and individual practitioners should be prepared to provide, or advocate, the services that are proving successful in demonstration projects.

FAMILY SUPPORT

When at all possible, the family (parents in most cases for young teenagers but occasionally a husband) rather than the service provider should be the first line of support for the adolescent. Some providers have a rescue fantasy. They want to help the pregnant teenager or young mother directly—to save her from her family.

This approach should only be used when there is strong evidence that the family's influence is a negative one, for example, that the family will be physically or emotionally abusive. A family whose members show ambivalence about a pregnant daughter should not be ignored. Such a family should be assisted to accept the adolescent and to adapt its activities to meet the new circumstances. This may involve individual or group counseling, home visits, and financial assistance.

Rather than work with an ambivalent family, some agencies find it easier to remove the youngster from her home and place her in an apartment of her own, with a foster family, or in a maternity home. But these solutions may not be effective in the long run. First, the adolescent parent will need, for an extended period, the many types of assistance a family can provide. If she is separated from her family during pregnancy or in the immediate postpartum period, she may have great difficulty in reestablishing the bond and thus be deprived of a future source of support.

Further, research has suggested that adolescents who continue to live with their families during their pregnancies and for several years afterward are more likely to continue school and to delay subsequent pregnancies. Benefits have also been shown for the child (Furstenberg and Crawford, 1978).

ADOLESCENTS AS PARENTS

Although the evidence is meager, it is generally assumed that pregnant teenagers do not usually become good mothers. Several reasons have been suggested for this assumption. First, they are too young. This is based on the belief that increased maturity or additional years of exposure to infants and young children will improve parenting skills. A second reason often cited is that the adolescent period itself is not suitable for parenting. The adolescent's search for independence conflicts with her needs for support as a mother and her infant's dependency. Limited formal education is another possible cause. Kinard and Reinherz (1983) found in a white working-class community that years of education had a greater effect than did maternal age on a child's psychological functioning in the early schoolyears. Finally, poverty may be the most significant reason for deficiencies in mothering. A large proportion of young parents are poor, and it is hard to be loving and to find time to stimulate and encourage a child's potential when obtaining food, clothing, and housing is a continuing struggle. (For a recent review of this subject, see Brooks-Gunn and Furstenberg, in press.)

Bierman and Street (1982) have described the problems that many teenagers face when they become parents. They urge service providers to address the adolescent needs of the young mothers as a first step in improving parenting skills: "Only after a teenager mother has dealt with her own needs, and has related her feelings to her child's, can she take the next step of providing consistent, empathic, ongoing care of her child."

Assuming that because of youth, lack of education, and poverty many young mothers have difficulty raising their children, providers need to find ways to prevent the emotional problems and low scores on intelligence tests that have been found in some studies. Kellam (1978, 1979) and others have suggested that the way to minimize these deficits is to make sure that the child has more than one adult caregiver.

Coletta (1981) demonstrated the impact on maternal behavior of social support from family and others. She found that the more support adolescent mothers received, the more affectionate they were to their children. Cuddling, comforting, and similar behaviors were more frequent in mothers who had high levels of support; those with little support were more likely to be rejecting, indifferent, or hostile. The most important source of support was the adolescent's family. In Coletta's words, "the adolescent's behavior was the most positively affected when she felt she had a close family which she could count on for help: when she felt that she could talk to her parents, when her parents treated her like an adult, and when there was no conflict over the way the adolescent was raising her child. Next in order of importance was emotional support from a partner or spouse." These findings provide additional reasons for strengthening the unmarried adolescent's family so that it will keep her at home: it will help the teenager's child avoid the problems often associated with being brought up by the mother alone or by the mother in company with another female adolescent, whether male or female.

STRENGTHENING SUPPORT NETWORKS

Zitner and Miller (1980) found that adolescent mothers were very dependent on informal support networks. Over three quarters of their study sample lived with their families. Not only did family members provide financial assistance, housing, clothing, food, and child care, but they also assisted in decision making. Few of the grandparents, however, reported receiving services from community agencies, and the researchers suggested that agencies try to strengthen the informal support system. They noted the conflicts that agencies can expect:

> Provision of services for the whole family is important, but professionals must not lose sight of the sometimes conflicting needs of family members. Many of the young mothers are still experiencing normal adolescent conflicts between dependency on their families and the desire to establish their independence. While the majority of the young mothers are dependent upon their families for the financial support and child-care assistance necessary to enable them to prepare themselves for self-sufficiency, they are, in many instances, eager to establish their own households. Service providers must work to enhance the strong informal support service network the family offers, while still recognizing and encouraging genuine and appropriate strivings for indepedence.

Several clinicians have described approaches to this dilemma of how to deal with both the adolescent and her family. Fine and Pape (1982) suggest a diagnostic process that will reveal family strengths and weaknesses leading to a matching of the adolescent's needs with her ecological networks (including her family of origin, extended family supports, and peer groups) and with the professional service network. Authier and Authier (1982) also urge that the service provider pay attention to the family when trying to assist the pregnant adolescent in making choices about her future. "Although the professional can choose to ignore the adolescent's family system, the adolescent will bring her family with her into treatment; if not in person, then as part of her framework for decision making, her learned pattern of response, and her understanding of herself and her situation."

Many programs across the United States attempt to provide support to families so that they can help adolescents through their pregnancies and the first few years of parenting. An example is the Prenatal and Early Infancy Project in Elmira, New York (Olds et al., 1983), which has as its goal the improvement of the conditions of pregnancy and early childrearing among high-risk families. Nurses visit study families twice a month beginning in the second trimester of pregnancy and continuing, with less frequency, through the second year of the baby's life. The program has three components: parent education, involvement of relatives and friends, and linkages with formal services. The investigators believe a mother's prenatal health habits and competence in early child care are related to the quality of her relations with others in her informal social environment. A key aspect of the home-visiting program consists of involving other family members or friends to whom the mother feels close. The nurse impresses upon these individuals the importance of proper diet, rest, exercise, and regular prenatal care as well as the dangers of smoking, drinking, and drugs. It is hoped that they will support the pregnant woman and the new mother in adopting positive physical and emotional health behaviors. (A list of similar programs can be found in *Programs to Strengthen Families*, assembled by the Yale Bush Center in Child Development and Social Policy.)

A THEORETICAL MODEL

Programs like these have in common an emphasis on assisting the pregnant adolescent and young mother directly, in working with her family or spouse so that these individuals may provide support, and in linking the adolescent and the family to community agencies that can provide more technical types of assistance. Perlman and Giele's (1983) Model of the Family Care System, although originally designed to help understand the role of the family in caring for elderly or disabled individuals, is equally useful in understanding the relation of the family and community resources to the needs of young mothers. The model describes an "unstable triad" with three variables: "1. the physical and emotional needs and demands that the dependent person places upon the family; 2. the material and non-material capacities of the families to meet the dependent person's needs and simultaneously to fulfill other family functions; and, 3. the availability and use of community resources such as social services."

Changes in any one of these components affects the others and should bring about compensatory adjustments. For example, if a pregnant adolescent living with her family is unable to continue caring for her infant when she returns to school, more caregiving will be needed from the family, friends, neighbors, or a daycare agency. Or if the grandmother who minds the baby decides to take a full-time job, the caring responsibilities will have to be shifted.

The model suggests how families may adjust to crises, first by exploring possible alternatives and then by trying methods of adjustment. The ultimate results are undoubtedly influenced by the family's experience with crisis management and problem resolution. Certain families cope more effectively with demands and crises and may be better able to care for a young mother and child than families with a less positive history.

Perlman and Giele point out the danger of exhausting family resources, including finances, time, and physical and emotional strength. If demands exceed the resources for a long time, "burn out" may occur and have a negative impact on the young mother and child. This should be avoided through counseling, financial support, daycare, and other services.

Conclusions

The importance of the family in providing support for the pregnant adolescent and the young mother has been noted clinically and confirmed by research. Nevertheless, there are situations in which the physical and emotional health of the young mother and her infant can only be ensured by removal from a family home, and communities must be prepared for such situations. Also family involvement should not include a requirement for parental notification or consent for birth-control services or abortions. Research has shown that assurance of confidentiality is one of the most important factors in teenagers' choice of a family-planning facility, and that they would be more reluctant to seek planning assistance if they knew their parents would be notified. (Zabin and Clark, 1983). Research has also shown that the Massachusetts law requiring parental or judicial consent for teenage abortions, while reducing the number of abortions within the state, has caused teenagers to seek this service elsewhere (Cartoof and Klerman, in press). Although parent-child communication about sexual activity, contraception, pregnancy, and childrearing should be encouraged, it is doubtful that it can be mandated by law.

Bearing children too early clearly places severe stress on adolescents, their families, and their infants. The first line of support to reduce such stress is the adolescent's family, but private providers and welfare agencies must also work to lighten the heavy burdens on both individuals and society of this major social problem.

V *

Policy Implications

$*$

FAMILY BREAKDOWN in divorce is rapidly increasing stresses on the families and children of our society. We must begin to take measures to prevent this breakdown, since the family is the most obvious system for achieving optimal developmental outcome in future generations. We must view it as a societal obligation to address the stresses on families and the supports needed to meet them. This also presents us with an opportunity to back up young families in a positive way at the time of organizing around a new baby or facing the normal problems of daily life. Helping young families learn to cope internally and to feel the rewards of coping successfully should become a major social goal. Many of our national policies reinforce failure and offer families little or no hope of improvement. It is time now to reinforce for strengths and coping systems that will reward individuals and their families. If we can build policies to support families as they learn to cope under normal developmental stress, they will be readier to cope with more unusual stresses, such as divorce and chronic illness.

Education in parenting as addressed by Bettye Caldwell offers us a chance to look at such a support system. Parents are feeling more empowered to seek what they need to be good parents. There is a body of information about child development which can help them do a better job. Middle- and upper-income parents are demanding it and will find ways to get it, regardless of cost. We need to find techniques to reach lower-income, more stressed parents. By considering education for parenting as just such an opportunity, we may indeed enable all parents to see parenthood as a rewarding experience.

Lisbeth Schorr, C. Arden Miller, and Amy Fine address which governmental policies have failed and which have succeeded in response to chronic stress during the past two economic recessions. We have given families some experience of societal support, and they may begin to demand it. So far, the United States is one of the last nations in the civilized world to make the needs of children and of families a priority. Despite protestations about caring for the family as an institution, the American government has cut back on major supportive policies. We have created a kind of hunger without the resources to match it. The inadequacy in government policy to support coping systems in intact families should be recognized as a missed opportunity to shore up society for the future. Grass-root movements should be encouraged to demand policy decisions that will support families in day-to-day coping as well as in crises. Otherwise, the future of our children and our society is endangered.

13 *

Education of Families
for Parenting

WITHOUT OUR BEING especially conscious of the transition, the word "parent" has gradually come to be used as much as a verb as a noun. Whereas we formerly thought mainly about "being a parent," we now find ourselves talking about learning how "to parent." This change, as is true of all language shifts, is undoubtedly very significant in terms of what it says about our perception of the essence of the role. It suggests that we may now be concentrating on action rather than status, on what we do rather than what or who we are.

Actually the words "mother" and "father" have always been used as verbs. In the limited etymological research I could do with the assortment of old and odd dictionaries lying around my study, I found only one that gave a verb form for "parent" and that meant "to originate or produce." Hardly what we are referring to when we talk about education for parenting! All of the dictionaries had both noun and verb forms for "mother" and "father," but, interestingly enough, they differed drastically in the breadth of action covered in the verb forms. Definitions for mother covered, in addition to birthing, such acts as "to care for or to protect like a mother." the verb definitions for father tended to be more limited and to cover mainly such functions as "to fix the paternity or origin of." Thus the use of "parent" as a verb—a trend about ten years old—is gradually developing the connotative meaning that is much closer to the verb form for mother than for father. In fact, the adoption of the word "parent" as a verb may be related to our increasing use of nongender terms and to our recognition of the overlap in roles played by mothers and fathers in the rearing of children. Certainly it is somehow based on our realization that the essence of parenting is less the determination of the origin of a child than the guidance of that child's continuous growth and development.

Brief History of the Field

Although we tend to think of parenting education as a relatively new phenomenon, this is not true. The Old Testament contains many admonitions for parents about the treatment of their children, as well as clear statements about some of the responsibilities of children (such as "Honor thy father and thy mother"). And, as would be expected, the ancient Greeks and only slightly more modern Romans had explicit codes (Caldwell, 1980). During the sixteenth century a few physicians who were especially concerned with children began to write materials intended for use by parents rather than writing exclusively for their professional colleagues. The best known of these are the Pediatric Poems discussed by John Ruhrah (1925).

Around the turn of the century in this country, the prestigious psychologist G. Stanley Hall freely wrote materials for parents. But the first well-known professional whose materials reached large numbers of parents was Arnold Gesell who, with his colleagues (Gesell and Ilg, 1943; Gesell and Amatruda, 1946), wrote a series of age- and stage-related books intended for parents and professionals alike. Then, in 1946, came the first edition of a parent-education manual that gained such wide acceptance and usage that its title was forgotten *(The Pocket Book of Baby and Child Care)* and it came instead to be known simply by the name of its author—Dr. Spock. During this same period, many magazines directed to parents were launched and gained impressive circulations as well as professional respect.

As other forms of mass media became available—radio, films, television—efforts were made to prepare interesting parent-education materials that would fit them. My own first professional assignment as a graduate student in child development consisted of preparing radio scripts for what the University of Iowa called the Radio Child Study Club. These were broadcast over the university radio station to community groups that had been organized all over the state (mainly by local PTA groups). The groups would meet in the home of one of the participants, listen to the program, and then discuss among themselves the materials covered in the script. Since I, at age twenty, wrote the scripts and prepared the discussion guides, I doubt that they got too much out of them. But it was an excellent idea—a unit of the extension service of the university, incidentally. Much parent-education work has been carried out over the years through cooperative extension programs in all the states.

Television has done less for parenting education than many feel it should have done. However, public education has certainly made some efforts in this area. During the 1979–80 season, a series of parent-education films called *Footsteps* was shown over public stations in most of the country. Various types of printed materials were available for follow-up activities. In Arkansas we bought a set of these tapes and used them in a unique way—to train foster mothers and family daycare mothers in principles of child development.

But education of families for parenting has not been totally dependent on the mass media. Churches, schools, parent-teacher organizations, clinics, health departments, child-care centers, and cooperative extension services have for years quietly carried on a campaign of trying to reach parents with either informational or emotional support which will in some way make their parenting task easier and more effective. Universities have been less involved in such activities than one might expect. Although professors in fields such as developmental psychology, family relations and child development, and early education have been strong proponents and have made themselves available as discussion leaders, official university sponsorship in the form of required or even elective classes has been minimal.

Thus we can say that education for parenting is not new, that its history has a fairly substantial conceptual and research substrate, and that we have now reached a point where there is almost a glut of materials on the market. Let me turn briefly to an examination of the underlying rationale for such efforts.

Rationale for Education

All such efforts at reaching parents have been based on a few simple yet profound assumptions. I can identify at least four.

The first assumption is that behavior is not determined entirely by the unfolding of certain "instincts" but is profoundly influenced by the exercise of knowledge and skills that can be acquired. Related to this is the assumption that parenting skills will show natural variation, just as any other human trait does, and that the important skills can be either acquired or improved with effort.

A second important underlying assumption that affects all programs is that parenting is an area in which a knowledge base exists pertaining to effective types of parenting behavior. Further, there is an apparent conviction that new knowledge develops through research and that even complex ideas can be "translated" into nonjargonized language that will register with any intelligent reader. Since the researchers themselves are not always the best translators of their ideas to people other than colleagues, this has given rise to a large number of middle persons (journalists, commentators, editorialists) who fulfill this vital translation role. Of course many of the professionals (such as Brazelton) remain their own best interpreters, but others, such as the late Jean Piaget, remain aloof to the task and seemingly indifferent to the translated products.

A third assumption that forms the rationale for such programs is that knowledge alone is not sufficient to develop parenting competence. That is, all major efforts at parenting education deal in some way with emotions and attitudes. Our basic ideas about how to parent are encrusted with deeply felt emotions and many myths. One of the myths of parenting is that it is always fun and games, joy and delight. Everyone who has been a parent will testify that it is also anxiety, strife, frustration, and even hostility. Thus most major parenting-education formats deal with parental emotions and attitudes and, to a greater or lesser extent, advocate that the emotional component is more important than the knowledge.

A final assumption is a very pragmatic one: everybody, no matter how well-educated or well-adjusted or well-mated, needs help in the parenting process. This need for help is presumably intensified by certain changes in today's living styles—fewer extended families offering grandmothers as experienced instructors, greater geographic mobility resulting in less extended family support even when separate households are maintained, smaller families who provide less opportunity to gain experience in caring for children while the parents themselves are growing up, and more very young parents who themselves have not been fully parented.

Program formats developed on the basis of this rationale have varied with the predilections of the developer. Many tend to be group-oriented, with strong feelings about the importance of contributions of other parents in the group as well as the input from the group leader. Although many leaders eschew a didactic approach, there is often some new informational input in most sessions. And certainly the programs have a strong "hands-on" component where possible. Programs offered in schools often combine sessions for the mothers and/or fathers with experience gained in observing trained child-care workers and possibly working with their own children in a child-care setting.

Many of the programs have tended to concentrate on two developmental periods—infancy and early childhood, and adolescence. Regardless of whether these periods warrant their reputation as more "difficult" developmentally, many parents seem more interested in and receptive to parenting programs when their children fall into these age groups.

Resistance to Education

In view of the reasonably respectable history of the field and the theoretically and empirically legitimate basis for parenting programs, it almost comes as a shock to realize just how intense the opposition to such efforts can be. It would be difficult to think of a preventive program with potentially greater payoff to society than the general improvement of parenting skills. Many of our expensive public health and public welfare programs—child abuse and neglect programs, residential and out-patient psychotherapy, rehabilitation following avoidable accidents, and so on—might be drastically curtailed if parents were more effective childrearers. And there has probably never been a time in history when more people were more vocal about the importance of the family to children and to society as a whole. Why, then, does one find such resistance to plans to make preparation for parenthood a regular part of our educational system?

Never was opposition more clamorous—and more effective— than at the White House Conference on Families (the conference, scheduled for 1980, actually took place in 1981, in part because of vehement opposition to such ideas as universal parent education). On the basis of comments made both by those who spoke at advance hearings and by some of the delegates, the main areas of resistance to parenting education included such things as:

— It was based on secular humanism and would destroy the spiritual values of the family.
— It would represent and encourage governmental intrusion into family life.
— It would encourage early and indiscriminate sexual experience and literally teach young people how to engage in such behavior.
— Under the protection of such terms as "values clarification" such courses would be teaching ethics and morals, which are the rightful prerogative of the family.
— It would be a waste of time because the "experts" don't agree with one another, and what is recommended in one decade is obsolete in the next.

In spite of these objections—and in spite of the vehemence and microphone-controlling procedures used in stating some of them— delegates attending all three of the regional conferences (Baltimore, Minneapolis, and Los Angeles) approved by large majorities the resolutions supporting family-life education. Recommendations made at the conferences had to be limited to one hundred words and were drafted by committees, conditions that do not always lead to perfect clarity of expression. Nonetheless, it is perhaps worth quoting the exact wording of three of the resolutions passed at the Los Angeles conference:

Parents, religious and ethnic groups, voluntary agencies, community organizations, and schools all have a legitimate and vital role in the lifelong process of developing and enriching marriage and family life. It is therefore recommended that both the public and private sector support family life programs, including required marriage preparation, human growth and development, responsible parenthood, effective communication, management of resources and skills necessary to produce them and making available family counseling. Personnel providing instruction and counseling in these areas should have adequate training and be able to demonstrate competency. [19th rank]

It shall be public policy that the primary responsibility for teaching preparation for parenthood and family life education lies with parents, who should be encouraged to teach it in the home. Such courses should be developed in local communities through the cooperation of parents, educators, professionals and religious leaders. These courses should be designed to teach parents who can effectively interpret, apply and personalize the training to the particular needs of their families. This does not preclude the development of other training programs, public or private. [26th rank]

The Federal Government should encourage states to provide comprehensive education for family life as a K-12 required curriculum in public schools. Such a curriculum should include, but not be limited to, communication and relationship skills, non-violent conflict resolution, decision-making, parenting and child care skills, health and nutrition, substance abuse prevention and human sexuality. Parents, teachers, students, community and church representatives should have the right to excuse a student from participating in any objectionable sections. Communities should be encouraged and assisted in offering continuing education and counseling in family life skills. [47th rank] (White House Conference, 1982)

All three of these resolutions—even the one pertaining to a role for the federal government—are mild and contain all sorts of safeguards specifying family input into curriculum and parental rights to ask that their children be excused from any "objectionable sections" of the units. Even so, support for any form of family-life education—the term that has come to be preferred over parenting education—was considerably watered down during the six-month implementation phase of the White House Conference. This was clearly a reflection of the organized opposition to such programs and the perception by conference staff that the issue was a political hot potato and should be dropped as quickly as possible.

Overcoming Resistance

In spite of this apparent official reduction of attention to the needs of young people for parenting education, and in spite of the presence of substantial numbers of opponents in most geographic regions, grassroots enthusiasm for such programs has grown steadily during the past five years all over the country. Dedicated people in many states are working systematically to facilitate the greater availability of such programs, particularly for the large numbers of young mothers who face childrearing responsibilities without a marital partner, without adequate economic resources, and often without biological family support and collaboration. In meeting with such groups, and in the process of helping to link one with another, I have been able to formulate several suggestions for making progress in the development of programs to help educate families for parenting. In the remainder of this chapter, I will summarize seven such suggestions.

1. Encourage the development of an historical orientation. Earlier I gave a brief history of parenting education. It is amazing to note how many people seem to think it is an entirely new venture, freshly devised to weaken the family. If we can inject into such accusations the reminder that parenting education in one form or another has been around for a long time and has played a respectable role in strengthening and preserving family life in America, this can help to make such assertions appear almost ridiculous. As cooperative extension programs are generally associated with other services to farm families, I always like to stress their role in the preparation and dissemination of parenting-education concepts. There is nothing more "mainline" and conservative than programs developed largely for rural America, and leaders of such programs have played extremely important roles in legitimizing and facilitating parenting programs. Likewise, most homes will have on the coffeetable one or more women's or home magazines, each of which will have one or more articles on some aspect of childrearing. Helping people who are afraid of such programs to realize that they have already endorsed them in one form or another can be a big help in overcoming opposition.

2. Appoint panels of parents to any curriculum committee relating to the development of a program for parenthood education.

You will recall that the wording of the resolution from the Los Angeles conference stressed the importance of this. Such panels should be created regardless of the planned auspices of the programs. The more "public and/or governmental" the program, however, the more important are such parent panels. This means that, as a curriculum committee is formed by a large public school district to work up a curriculum for secondary students, the committee should contain several parents in addition to the teachers, supervisors, and principals who generally make up such committees. Efforts should be made to see to it that all such meetings are open and that visitors are welcome. Once written, curricula should be available for scrutiny and study. Abbreviated workshops to allow parents to take a minicourse using the materials prepared for the courses would be helpful. If the committee is choosing rather than developing a curriculum, then parents should have a vote in the selection process. Such openness will make allies of parents rather than potential enemies.

3. If necessary, omit sex education from the curriculum. Since many people consider sex education one of the most important components of a parenting-education curriculum, this may appear to be a cowardly capitulation. I would disagree. The concepts of responsible parenting can undoubtedly best be dealt with in a curriculum that also involves responsible sexuality. But there is so great a need for other components in education for parenthood that it is foolish to allow this one area of resistance to block needed programs.

Various communities have devised different techniques for dealing with resistance to sex education. In Kentucky, where parenting courses are offered in the public schools, parents must give permission for their adolescent children to participate in the sex-education unit. If parents withhold such permission, a set of the teaching materials to be used is sent home and the parents are asked to cover the materials with their children themselves. This is a beautifully adaptive procedure—undoubtedly better than leaving the unit out or shutting the course down altogether because of the objections of one or two parents.

Scales (1981) reminds us that people who object to sex education have legitimate concerns and should not be dealt with in a knee-jerk denunciation:

Sex education proponents must recognize that not all opponents are extremists who threaten democratic traditions; many in fact have raised reasonable questions regarding teacher training, values, age-appropriateness of content, and the use of certain materials that can, if genuinely considered, greatly improve the education we offer. Yet, when those concerns are facilely dismissed as the grumblings of a "lunatic fringe," we both lose the opportunity for improvement and invite the ire of those people whom we have disrespectfully cast aside. (p. 565)

4. Consider the possibilities for infusion of parenting education rather than addition of a new subject to the curriculum. When one advocates such courses in junior high and high schools, one is usually met with a moaning question, "But what would we take out? The schedule is already overloaded!" This is a legitimate complaint. Yet it is not necessary to add a new course or subject in order to cover most of the topics dealt with in preparation for parenthood classes. Topics that need to be covered in such classes are dealt with, either directly or indirectly, in a number of subject areas already securely ensconced in the curriculum at all grade levels. For example, many health-education units already have some sort of unit on human biology, including reproduction. Birth control can easily be included in such units. Social-studies classes at all levels deal with the family as a basic social unit and often get into areas such as family conflict and family variants (one-parent families, reconstituted families, and so on). Furthermore, in literature there are many great novels and short stories, quite likely to be on required reading lists, which provide opportunities for exploration of feelings and the acquisition of new knowledge pertaining to child development.

To give an example of this, at an elementary school where I once served as principal (in Little Rock, Arkansas), we built the entire curriculum for a six-week period around Charles Dickens' *Oliver Twist* and the musical *Oliver!* A children's version was used as a reader with the older (grades 4 and 5) children. Math problems were written that dealt in some way with the story: "If a loft contains 645 square feet and if 12 orphans and 1 man live there, how many square feet per person are there in the loft?" Many of the art projects during the period pertained to the story. The upper-level children improvised a loft in the upstairs hall of the school and populated it with papier-maché orphans whom they dressed in their own clothes. The story was a natural for social studies at all levels: Why were there so many orphans at that time? Why did so many mothers die in childbirth? Why would a mother who had a child when she was not married want to die? Would this happen today? What kind of personality does a child develop who has no one to love or who was never loved by a parent? How could a criminal like Fagin keep the boys under his control? How did the boys learn to get along with one another? Where were the girl orphans? What kinds of social programs do we have for such children today? Do they all become criminals? What role does a father (or substitute) play in a child's development? How did Oliver develop a conscience? Obviously, the possibilities are endless and are adaptable to all grade levels. Our unit was climaxed by a school version of the musical, which, I assure you, did not leave a dry eye in the house. (For another example of an effective child-development unit in a public school, see Children, videotape.)

5. Encourage colleges and universities to consider courses in parenting. As I indicated earlier, our colleges have done little in this area other than supply dedicated professors who participate in such programs elsewhere. The big push today is to develop more and more programs for high schools and even junior highs because of the increasing number of births to teenage mothers. Such an emphasis is entirely appropriate. However, there is no justification for not planning more such programs—and requiring them of students—at the college level. University endorsement of an idea does, in our society, carry a certain status. Now it is as though curriculum committees in most universities do not consider such programs sufficiently "heavy" or intellectual to warrant their inclusion in the undergraduate requirements. Again, such materials can be easily infused into existing courses (psychology, sociology, child development). The main advantage to courses that are clearly labeled as education for parenting (under whatever name is currently popular) is that such labeling carries the imprimatur of the university and signifies public acceptance of the courses as important and worthwhile.

6. Try to build a case for the practical advantages of developing more competent parents. Most of us have a tendency to oversell

new programs in which we believe deeply, and it is possible that we are currently overselling the value of education for parenting. At least implicitly, if not in actual words, we offer to help prevent child abuse, improve mental health, decrease intrafamily strife, optimize children's development. These are essentially quasi-happiness outcomes. While we hope for such results, we may be better off to stress even seemingly trivial financial savings associated with such programs. In this regard, we would do well to take cognizance of what Lazar and Darlington (1982) and Weikart and his colleagues (Berrueta-Clement, 1984) have done regarding the long-term effects of early childhood programs. That is, they have stressed the economic savings associated with participation in such programs through fewer special-education assignments and grade repetitions. Those of us who advocate courses in education for parenting might do well to emulate this approach and suggest that such services can play an important role in the minimization of expensive rehabilitative and therapeutic programs.

7. Stress the consensual nature of the content of most parent-education programs. As mentioned earlier, a frequent derisive objection to such programs is that we don't know what to teach in them. This represents lack of conviction that we truly have a body of basic knowledge substantial enough to support practical applications. On the other hand, some opponents seem to fear a Machiavellian conspiracy to teach ideas that would subvert family and religious values. It is as though they fear that basic knowledge which would allow this is indeed available and all too easy to apply.

It is my conviction that there is indeed a sufficient body of knowledge available to allow such courses to be planned. Furthermore, it is almost inconceivable that the core ideas could be objectionable to anyone—conservative, middle-of-the-road, or liberal. Such curricula stress such things as the overwhelming importance of the parent in a child's life, the importance of love and the way it develops in daily life, the responsibilities and rights of parents, the importance of providing early and appropriate stimulation and of responding to the infant's own behavior, the value of toys and play materials, and the needs of infants for stability and predictability in people and events. Most programs offer opportunities for practical experience with young children, a feature that many regard as the most valuable aspect of the training. Participants are given an opportunity to learn to recognize developmental milestones and to expect and deal with individual differences in children, to know the health and nutritional needs of young children, and to acquire skills in disciplining without physical punishment. Communications with parents regarding these general goals and strategies of education will generally provide reassurance to parents that their own values will be strengthened, not contradicted, by such training.

Summary

In this chapter I have reflected on the meaning for us of the increasingly common usage of the word "parent" as a verb, have offered a brief history of efforts to provide family education for parenting, have presented what can be deduced as the underlying rationale for such programs, and have described some of the patterns of resistance to them. Finally I have offered seven suggestions of ways to defuse this resistance. At this point in history we need simply to move ahead in the task, aware of deep differences in perceptions of the reality of the field between groups characterized as the "right" and the "left," and equally aware that we are not likely to be able to reconcile all these differences at the present time. However, by being open in our planning and in our program operation, by drawing circles that take opponents in rather than keep them out, and by stressing the consensual nature of our core curriculum, we can nonetheless move ahead.

LISBETH B. SCHORR,
C. ARDEN MILLER, and
AMY FINE

14 ✱

The Social-Policy Context
for Families Today

It is clear that current arrangements for distributing responsibility for our young between family and community are in turmoil. Past arrangements are plainly out of kilter with present and future needs. Social and demographic changes have combined to diminish the likelihood that families can assure their children's healthy growth and development without help from outside the family—at the very time that there is growing skepticism about the desirability and workability of societal action to provide the supports that families require.

Because recent social changes have occurred so rapidly, our problems today may be considerably more acute than those faced by previous generations and other societies. Many of those who must decide about the allocation of resources and the proper role of government at various levels grew up in an age when the rules, the resources, and the problems were markedly different from what they are today. Legislators ask how *their* mothers managed without the government programs they are asked to support. Why can't the mothers of today do the same? Why do they have to be coddled? Why do they require continually increasing appropriations to maternal and child health programs or Medicaid, while yesterday's mothers had to manage on their own.

Two points are crucial in understanding the changes that have occurred since previous generations came of age. First, today it is possible to help in ways that were undreamed of earlier in this century. Fewer babies die during the first year of life. Death in childbirth has been virtually eliminated, as have deaths due to diphtheria, whooping cough, and measles. Life expectancy has increased by nearly two decades since the beginning of the century. That modern medicine and public health can accomplish so much is of course a fact to be celebrated. Yet it also results in higher costs, and in more troublesome and difficult policy decisions, because the stakes in how society distributes the benefits have grown accordingly.

Second, for earlier generations, in one way or another there were more adults in and around the family to provide children with caring, nurturance, and guidance. There were more two-parent families, more extended families living together or in close proximity, and far fewer families where both parents worked. The family's ability to rear and protect children was threatened and often severely compromised by the Great Depression. But we learned from those years and enacted new legislation to protect families and individuals against some of the most devastating effects of unemployment, old age, disability, and death. We provided specified populations, especially poor mothers and children, with certain minimal health services. Increasing economic prosperity and a second wave of social legislation in the mid-1960s served in some measure to buffer the growing stresses of changing family structures and rapidly increasing mobility.

Today, however, the number of children in circumstances of high risk—for social or economic reasons—is increasing, while the availability of formal social supports is decreasing.

— More than one fifth of all American children live with only one parent. (Select Panel, 1981)
— Since 1977, the majority of American mothers have been working. Since 1983, the majority of mothers with children under six have been working. And today nearly half of all mothers with children under three are in the labor force. (Bureau of Labor Statistics, 1983; Kammerman, 1984)
— National unemployment figures are down to 7.8 percent from a December 1982 high of just below 11 percent, but ten states, with a combined population of more than 40

million, still have unemployment rates of over 11.5 percent. Bureau of Labor Statistics, 1983)

— The teenage jobless rate was a record 24.5 percent at the end of 1982, with black teenage unemployment close to 50 percent. (Cummings, 1983a)

— High rates of unemployment among black men of all age groups has had a particularly devastating impact on black families. A 1983 *New York Times* survey of black women found that while each woman's story was different, the most common thread among those heading families alone "was the inability of the fathers of their children to hold steady jobs" (Cummings, 1983b). Today, while the official unemployment rate for black males is 18 percent, this figure may seriously underestimate the true rate of joblessness among blacks, since it does not include those not actively looking for work and those omitted from the 1980 census (Bureau of Labor Statistics, 1984). A study by the Center for the Study of Social Policy estimates that only 54 percent of all black men are actually working (Joe and Yu, 1984). Thus it is not surprising that 42 percent of black families are single-parent, female-headed families. (CSSP, 1984b)

The impact on children of unemployment and changing family structure is compounded by unequal patterns of income distribution. The United States probably has the most unequal income distribution of any Western industrialized nation. Budget cuts and changes in the tax structure enacted in 1981 have made the rich still richer and the poor still poorer, so that today the poorest fifth of the American population receives 4.2 percent of the national income, while the richest fifth receives 43 percent, or more than ten times as much (Havemann, 1982).

In terms of setting policy, the most important fact to understand about children growing up in the United States today is that so many of them are poor. The proportion of children living in poverty, which had fallen to 14 percent in 1969, rose to 21.3 percent in 1982 (U.S. Congress, 1983). In just two years, between 1981 and 1983, the number of children living in poverty increased by two and a half million. And while poverty is not in itself a deterrent to normal development, it is, in the words of Albert J. Solnit, a "major medium in which high-risk environments are cultured."

The trends that seem to account for large and growing numbers of children in poverty are high unemployment and what has come to be called the "feminization" of poverty: the great increase in the number of households headed by women, with women's lower incomes and high expenses for child care. The Congressional Budget Office projects no decline in the proportion of children living in poverty during the years immediately ahead, even if other indicators of recession improve (Rivlin, 1983).

Nevertheless, many of the social and health services that could protect families and children from some of the adverse effects of recessions and high unemployment rates have, over the past several years, been cut back and eroded. Many of these programs and services were far from adequate at their best; some needed reform, some needed expansion, some needed to be better coordinated with other programs. (It is one of the minor ironies of history that a blueprint for action to strengthen national child health policy, requested by Congress in 1979 and carefully designed and documented by the Select Panel for the Promotion of Child Health in the ensuing two years, was never seriously considered by Congress. The 1981 agendas of neither advocates nor legislators allowed room for consideration of the fundamental reforms proposed by the panel.)

Over the past several years, programs for children were not cut as deeply as originally proposed by the Reagan Administration, thanks to the extraordinary efforts of a large number of dedicated individuals and highly effective advocacy organizations. The Children's Defense Fund, the Food Research and Action Center, and professional organizations, including the American Academy of Pediatrics and the American Public Health Association, worked successfully to minimize the damage by mobilizing the reservoir of fairness and caring that clearly still exists in this country. Still, supports for children and their families through Medicaid, maternal and child health programs, AFDC, nutrition programs, day-care and child protection services—many of which were shockingly underfunded in the past—have been further weakened over the last few years, not only by monetary cutbacks but also by assaults on the very structures on which these programs were built. Preventive services of all kinds have been particularly hard hit and often abandoned.

In the Medicaid program, cutbacks of $3.1 billion in federal funding since 1981 have deepened the impact of reduced family incomes and loss of health insurance. One study shows that the number of Americans without health insurance increased by 9.9 million between 1979 and 1982, in part because of unemployment and in part because changing employer attitudes toward health insurance led many companies to drop family coverage (Swartz, 1984).

Compounding the effect of reductions in Medicaid, federal funds for maternal and child health were cut by 18 percent in 1982. In 1983, the Congress increased MCH funding as part of the Emergency Assistance Jobs Bill, but current funding is still 16 percent below the amounts needed to maintain 1980 real purchasing power (Allen, 1983).

In 1982, forty-seven states cut back their MCH services or reduced eligibility. Forty-four states made these cuts by reducing prenatal and delivery services for pregnant women, and primary and preventive health care for infants, children, and women of childbearing age. Twenty-seven states achieved savings by cutting services for handicapped children (Allen, 1983).

With regard to income assistance, the most important thing to remember is that in *no* state today do AFDC benefits, even in combination with food stamps, allow families dependent on these programs an income as high as the officially established poverty level (U.S. Congress, 1983).

As for nutrition programs, the food-stamp program has been drastically cut since 1981. One million people, many of them children, have had their eligibility for food stamps terminated, and about 4 million have had their benefits reduced. Other nutrition programs, especially the school-lunch program, have been similarly curtailed (Greenstein, 1983).

Cutbacks in child welfare and other social service programs, including a 21 percent decrease in funding for the Social Services Block Grant, have left many struggling families with no place to go for help (Allen, 1983). Preventive services, so crucial to avoiding dependency, unwarranted out-of-home placements, and high and often unnecessary long-range costs, have been virtually eliminated in many states. Child protection agencies report significant increases in need and demand for services, while the availability of support services has decreased or remained constant in about three quarters of the agencies.

Forty-two states have made changes that threaten to lower the quality of child-care services, by cutting back on the training of workers, quality monitoring, or support services to care providers, and by lowering their care standards (Blank 1983).

To make judgments about the impact of the policy changes and funding cutbacks just described, we need information about ultimate outcomes for the families and children who are affected. It is particularly important to assess these program and policy changes in terms of what they have meant for the actual health and well-being of children in the light of suggestions that cutbacks have simply resulted in the elimination of inefficiencies and duplications. Our ability to measure ultimate outcomes for families and children, especially in the subtle and complex areas of psychosocial development, is limited. Even in the areas of physical health, where measurement is easier, we have—with some notable exceptions—an imperfect understanding of the causal connections between services and outcomes.

Despite the limitations of both our data and our ability to make accurate policy inferences from what we know, policy decisions must be made. It is therefore imperative, especially in this era of rapid change, that we scrutinize thoroughly and thoughtfully what information we have, so that policy making will be based as fully as possible on solid information and analysis.

The main conclusion from a review of what we know about outcomes for American children today is that, while in general they are getting healthier, there are causes for alarm, which suggest that the institutions serving children and families are failing in some very significant ways. First, several important health indicators show substantial and, in some instances, increasing disparities between the general population and major racial and socioeconomic subgroups. Second, other measures of well-being suggest that certain outcomes that indicate damage to young people also threaten the health, integrity, and future productivity of the entire society.

Disparities in Health Status

To provide a sense of the problem of disparities in health status between the general population and more vulnerable subgroups, we consider three indicators: infant mortality, low birth weight, and nutritional deficiencies.

INFANT MORTALITY

Infant mortality rates (IMRs) are the most familiar traditional indicator of the health and welfare of populations and subpopulations. In the United States the IMR has been fairly steadily declining since the beginning of the century, reflecting increasing access to adequate sanitation, food, shelter, education, and health services.

This encouraging picture changes when one looks more closely at especially vulnerable populations. Some states and cities with high unemployment rates, low per-capita income, and large minority populations have experienced a leveling off of previously favorable trends—or even an increase in IMR. Whether one looks at trends over the past five years or the past twenty, at hard-hit states or the entire nation, the gap between black and white IMRs not only continues but is increasing (Sanders, 1984).

LOW BIRTH WEIGHT

In the United States the proportion of babies born at low weight is one of the highest among industrialized nations. At the same time, Americans have the best record for weight-specific survival. Our high infant mortality rate is due largely to the high proportion of low-birth-weight babies. These infants are at greater risk not only of dying in their first year but of mental retardation, birth defects, growth and developmental problems, visual and hearing defects, delayed speech, learning problems, and even abuse and neglect.

Currently, close to 7 percent of all births in the United States are classified as low-weight. Since 1980, there has been no improvement in this overall figure (NCHS, Natality, 1983). Some urban areas have actually experienced increases. These included Atlanta, Detroit, New Orleans, and Richmond, among others.

Black babies are over twice as likely as white babies to be low in birth weight. In the past decade, the black/white ratio for low birth weight has increased from 2.03 to 2.19 in the United States (NCHS, Health, 1983).

ANEMIA AND GROWTH STUNTING

Both anemia and growth stunting reflect access to food, services, and supports necessary to resist infection and maintain adequate growth and development. The 1970s witnessed an enormous growth in supplemental food and nutrition programs, and by the late 1970s reports indicated that hunger and serious undernutrition had dramatically declined. More recent reports, however, are disquieting. To cite just two examples: In Boston, three times the expected rate of children admitted to Boston City Hospital's emergency room were found to be below the lowest 5th percentile for growth (Brown, 1983). In Massachusetts as a whole, health officials estimate that 10,000 to 17,500 low-income preschool children are chronically undernourished (Massachusetts, 1983).

Additional Measures of Health and Well-being

A second set of indicators, including drug and alcohol abuse, early teenage pregnancy, child abuse, and school failure are particularly troublesome, both because some of them are more difficult to define and keep track of and because the means of preventive intervention are even less clearly understood. At the same time, these indicators often reflect long-term problems, in which society's stake is enormous.

DRUG AND ALCOHOL ABUSE

While there has been some decline in teenage drug use in the United States in recent years, present levels of illicit drug use are still the highest in any industrialized nation. Adolescent use of alcohol, cigarettes, and other drugs is of major concern, in part because drugs and alcohol are involved in an extremely high proportion of violent deaths among young people and because of the impact of their use on emotional, cognitive, and physical development during this highly vulnerable period of growth.

One in nineteen high-school seniors reports drinking alcohol daily, a similar number smokes marijuana daily, and 41 percent engage in "binge drinking." Use of these substances begins at increasingly earlier ages. Three out of five marijuana and inhalant users had their first experience with these drugs between the sixth and ninth grades (Metropolitan, 1984).

TEENAGE CHILDBEARING

Early teenage childbearing, which is more common in the United States than in almost any other industrialized nation, is likely to prevent young women from completing their high-school education and becoming self-supporting. Their babies are at significantly increased risk of low birth weight, death in the first year, congenital defects, handicapping conditions, and learning problems.

CHILD ABUSE AND NEGLECT

The occurrence of child abuse and neglect represents a breakdown in the ability of a family (or of the larger society when a child is being cared for outside the home) to protect, nurture, and support a child, reflecting the need for a wide range of measures that reduce the risk from individual, family, and social conditions associated with maltreatment. There is increasing evidence of the profound and long-term physical and emotional consequences of child abuse and neglect.

Both state and individual agencies report increases in the number of referrals for child protective services, in the severity of injuries they are seeing, and in the multiplicity and chronicity of the client problems they are encountering. Child abuse is reported by many observers to be especially high in homes with unemployed parents (Coolsen, 1982).

SCHOOL FAILURE

School are not succeeding in educating our young in ways that are commensurate with society's needs. Why schools are failing in their educational mission is hotly debated and not well understood. Among the reasons may be factors intrinsic to the way schools themselves function, the possibility that too many students are entering school inadequately prepared for formal learning, and the absence of support for learning in the home and community environments.

The high-school dropout rate is 27 percent nationally and near 40 percent in many major American cities. Minorities are disproportionately affected by school failure. In a 1980 national representative sample of eighteen- to twenty-three-year-olds, seven of every hundred were found to lack the minimum vocational aptitude required for entry into the armed forces, including 26 percent of blacks and 20 percent of Hispanics of both sexes (Bock, 1981).

Supports To Improve Outcomes

This depressing litany should not lead to despair, for there is a solid basis for both optimism and action. The available evidence makes it quite clear that support from outside the family, in the form of income supplements, employment-related benefits, health, nutritional and social services, and more effective schools and preparation for school can protect against, or at least cushion, the effects of adverse environmental circumstances. The evidence for this conclusion comes from a wide array of sources, including an analysis of the contrasting effects of two recent recessions and evaluations of a variety of specific interventions and institutional changes.

EFFECTS OF TWO RECESSIONS

First there is the evidence from the recession of the mid-1970s. We now know that growing service programs did in fact protect children against some of the effects of that recession. During 1974–75, monthly unemployment rates reached 9.2 percent, rivaling those of 1981–82. But throughout the 1970s the exercise of public responsibility for financing and providing essential services and supports held constant or was expanded. Unemployment benefits were maintained at a high level, and benefits under Medicaid, AFDC, food stamps, and the WIC program were actually increased. As an apparent consequence, most measures of health status and health risks for children, including infant mortality, low birth weight, receipt by pregnant women of early prenatal care, and evidence of hunger and malnutrition, showed steady improvement throughout the 1970s, even among populations of states that were hardest hit by recession (Miller, 1983).

These findings have led us to conclude that public supports and services during the recession of 1974–75 effectively mitigated the adversities of unemployment and impoverishment, protecting children from some of the worst effects of a serious temporary recession and of increasing rates of poverty.

Children were not similarly protected against the recession of 1981–82, when many public health and social programs that had been working effectively were curtailed. Outcome data, some of which were reviewed above, indicate that children, families, and the society as a whole were subjected to serious and preventable risks and damage. Our findings strongly suggest that when either local or widespread economic reversals are anticipated, health services and social supports for children need to be expanded, not contracted.

EFFECTIVENESS OF PRENATAL CARE

The receipt of prompt and adequate prenatal care is strongly associated with infant survival and healthy development, especially for very young, poor, unmarried, or minority mothers who are at increased risk of poor pregnancy outcome. It has been shown quite clearly, by studies conducted in Ohio, California, Georgia, Texas, and Rhode Island, that better pregnancy outcomes for disadvantaged groups is a realistic goal, that it can be achieved by making appropriate services more widely available, and that it saves money (Miller, 1983).

There is good reason to believe that the increase in infant mortality and low birth weight currently becoming apparent among disadvantaged subpopulations is related at least in part to declines in the receipt of first-trimester prenatal care among vulnerable young women.

Preschool Interventions

A third example that demonstrates that poor outcomes are not the inexorable consequence of high-risk beginnings is the evidence of effectiveness of interventions during infancy and the preschool period. Because so many new systematic intervention programs were initiated in the second half of the 1960s, some of which included careful longitudinal studies, we are just beginning to learn of the strength and sturdiness of the long-term effects of these early interventions.

As a stellar example, the Yale Child Welfare Research Program, under the leadership of Sally Provence, provided a diverse and flexible cluster of intensive, clinically oriented services in homes and in a center to infants and their families. At five- and ten-year follow-up, participating families were significantly more upwardly mobile than control groups, including greater educational advancement, economic self-sufficiency, a lower birth rate, and improved "quality of life." Participating children had improved school attendance and better vocabulary than controls, and participating boys needed fewer special school services than controls (Rescorla, Provence, and Naylor 1982; Trickett et al., 1982).

In home-visiting programs in Montreal, Denver, and Appalachia, visited families had some combination of fewer home accidents, fewer problems with feeding and mother-child interactions, reduced incidence of child abuse, more up-to-date immunizations, and scored higher on assessments of home environments and maternal behavior (Select Panel, 1981).

Studies of the long-term effects of Headstart and other group preschool programs, especially those with significant parent participation, show similarly encouraging findings. One of the Headstart programs that has been particularly assiduous in pursuing followup data is the Perry Preschool Project of Ypsilanti, Michigan. There David Weikart and his colleagues found, in recent followup to age nineteen, that participants—in comparison with controls—had significantly lower rates of delinquency, lower numbers of pregnancies, higher scores on the Adult Performance Test, and included a higher number of high-school graduates (Schweinhart and Weikart, 1980; Berreuta-Clement et al., 1983).

In Brookline, Massachusetts, the most recently published results of the Early Education Project tell a similar story, pointing once more to the key role of parent involvement in early intervention and demonstrating that a comprehensive program with aggressive outreach to families with limited educational backgrounds clearly increases the proportion of children who attain competency standards, and that even in purely economic terms the returns on the investment far outweigh the costs (Pierson, Walker, and Tivnan, 1984).

As documented results like these begin to accumulate, and the public is made increasingly aware of them, there seems to be more hope of modifying the prevailing despair about the possibility of effective interventions to prevent the most damaging effects of adverse social and economic circumstances.

The Need To Act on What We Know

There are many more examples of demonstrably effective interventions. We have the knowledge, to a much greater extent than is commonly recognized, to make the institutions that are supposed to serve children and their families responsive to their most urgent needs. We must act on that knowledge. At the neighborhood, community, and state levels we must change the operations of schools, preschools, daycare, health services, social agencies, welfare, and job programs. We cannot continue allowing them to go without the funds, commitment, and talents necessary to do what must be done to fulfill the nation's obligations to its families and children.

We know and can readily demonstrate that services need to be sustained to be effective, that no single intervention or period of intervention will be a panacea. Appropriate interventions must be available at all stages of a child's development; no one intervention will "immunize" children or their families against harmful outcomes. We know and can demonstrate that help to individuals and families in trouble is more effective when the source of help includes a capacity for providing concrete and flexible assistance. Often this involves reaching around traditional agency procedures and traditional concepts of professionalism.

Private industry, together with government, can take long-overdue steps to help us catch up with European countries in our arrangements to provide maternity and infant-care leaves. Few modern societies go as far as ours in asking women to barter the welfare of their newborns for their own economic or professional survival.

At the national level, there must be greater recognition of the costs of *not* providing needed help. As today's children grow to adulthood, they will have to perform increasingly complex tasks, in an age of constant technological change, in order to protect the natural environment, uphold the standard of living, keep the economy competitive with other nations, maintain humanitarian values and—yes—preserve the nation's defense capabilities. Improving the health and well-being of today's children not only enhances the quality of their lives now; it also expands their potential to make significant contributions as adults.

More Americans must come to understand that their government spends less on social welfare, health insurance, child care, education, and unemployment benefits than governments of most other industrialized nations, leaving a greater share of the burden on individual families. In the United States in 1980, government spending at all levels and for all purposes, including national defense, amounted to a smaller proportion of gross national product than did public expenditures in Austria, Belgium, Canada, Denmark, France, Italy, the Netherlands, Norway, Sweden, the United

Kingdom, and West Germany (Miller and Schorr, 1983). It is hard to believe that this nation has achieved an optimal balance between private and public good at the present time.

Early in his administration, and only eight years after leading the Allied armies to victory in Europe, President Eisenhower told the American Society of Newspaper Editors,

> Every gun that is made, every warship launched, every rocket fired signifies . . . a theft from those who hunger and are not fed, those who are cold and are not clothed. This world in arms is not spending money alone. It is spending the sweat of its laborers, the genius of its scientists, the hope of its children. (CDF, 1984)

It is essential to recognize that public policy, which owes much to sound evidence, owes even more to societal values. In the last several years we have seen profound changes in public policy, not based on new and better data but growing out of an ideology that is rooted in the conviction that great societal benefits derive from accumulated wealth and military might. Bold actions have been taken to promote these ends in the name of coping with an economic crisis and a presumed national security crisis.

But we may be facing a different kind of crisis, involving human values. People who are knowledgeable about children and families, and the circumstances that cause them to flourish, must help in restoring to this nation's prevailing values a commitment to community, to shared responsibility, to caring for each other in both private and public settings, so that we may guide our children in directions that are promising for them as well as for the society that nurtures and is nurtured by them.

References

Introduction

Ashby, R. 1956. *An introduction to cybernetics*. London: Chapman and Hall.

Bertalanffy, L. von. 1968. *General systems theory*. New York: Braziller.

Bowlby, J. 1969. *Attachment and loss*, vol. 1, *Attachment*. New York: Basic Books.

Cannon, W. 1930. Organization for physiological homeostasis. *Physiological Review* 9:399.

Coles, R. 1985. *The moral life of children*. Boston: Atlantic Monthly Press.

Konner, M. 1982. *The tangled wing*. New York: Harper and Row.

Minuchin, S. 1974. *Families and family therapy: a structural approach*. Cambridge: Harvard University Press.

Patterson, G. R. 1983. Stress: a change agent for family process. In N. Garmezy and M. Rutter, eds., *Stress, coping and development in children*. New York: McGraw Hill.

Sander, L. W. 1977. The regulation of exchange in the infant-caretaker system and some aspects of the context-content relationship. In M. Lewis and L. Rosenblum, eds., *Interaction, conversation and the development of language*. New York: Wiley.

Vaillant, G. 1977. *Adaptation to life*. Boston: Little Brown.

Yogman, M. W. 1982. Development of the father-infant relationship. In H. Fitzgerald, B. Lester, and M. Yogman, eds., *Theory and research in behavioral pediatrics*, vol. 1. New York: Plenum Press.

—— 1983. Fathers' roles with children and youth: present at birth, discouraged thereafter? Testimony before U.S. Congress, House Select Committee on Children, Youth and Families. Economic Security Task Force, November 10, 1983, Washington, D.C.

1. Family Systems

Author's note: Figure 5, from Reiss and Costell (1977, p. 22), is reprinted by permission of The American Psychiatric Association, copyright 1977.

Bluebond-Langner, M. 1978. *The private worlds of dying children.* Princeton: Princeton University Press.

Costell, R., D. Reiss, H. Berkman, and C. Jones. 1981. The family meets the hospital: predicting the family's perception of the treatment program from its problem solving style. *Archives of General Psychiatry* 38:569–577.

Oliveri, M., and D. Reiss. 1981. A theory-based empirical classification of family problem solving behavior. *Family Process* 20:409–418.

Reiss, D. 1981. *The family's construction of reality.* Cambridge: Harvard University Press.

——— and R. Costell. 1977. The multiple family group as a small society: family regulation of interaction with nonmembers. *American Journal of Psychiatry* 134:21–24. Fig. 5

——— R. Costell, C. Jones, and H. Berkman. 1980. The family meets the hospital: a laboratory forecast of the encounter. *Archives of General Psychiatry* 37:141–154.

——— and D. Klein. Forthcoming. Paradigm and pathogenesis. In J. Theodore, ed., *Family interaction and psychopathology: theories, methods and findings,* New York: Plenum Press.

——— S. Gonzalez, and N. Kramer. Forthcoming. Family process, chronic illness and death. *Archives of General Psychiatry.*

Steinglass, P., S. Temple, S. Lisman, and D. Reiss. 1982. Coping with spinal cord injury: the family objective. *General Hospital Psychiatry* 4:259–264.

——— L. Bennett, S. Wolin, and D. Reiss. Forthcoming. *The alcoholic family.* New York: Basic Books.

Wynne, L. 1984. The epigenesis of relational systems: a model for understanding family development. *Family Process* 3:297–318.

2. Psychosocial Stress in Children

Author's note: Preparation of this chapter was supported in part by the John D. and Catherine T. MacArthur Foundation.

Barron, A., and F. Earls. 1984. The relation of temperament and social factors to behavior problems in three-year-old children. *Journal of Child Psychology and Psychiatry* 25:23–33.

Beautrais, A. L., D. M. Fergusson, and F. T. Shannon. 1982. Life events and childhood morbidity: a prospective study. *Pediatrics* 70:935–940.

Burke, J. D., J. F. Borus, B. J. Burns, et al. 1982. Changes in children's behavior after a natural disaster. *American Journal of Psychiatry* 139:1010–14.

Chess, S., A. Thomas, S. Korn, et al. 1983. Early parental attitudes, divorce and separation, and young adult outcome: findings from a longitudinal study. *Journal of the American Academy of Child Psychiatry* 22:47–51.

Earls, F. 1980. The prevalence of behavior problems in three year old children: a cross-national replication. *Archives of General Psychiatry* 37:1153–57.

———— 1982. Cultural and national differences in the epidemiology of behavior problems of preschool children. *Culture, Medicine and Psychiatry* 6:45–56.

———— 1983. An epidemiological approach to the study of behavior problems in very young children. In S. B. Guze, F. J. Earls, and J. E. Barrett, eds., *Childhood psychopathology and development.* New York: Raven Press.

———— E. Smith, and W. Reich. Submitted for publication. Psychopathological consequences of a disaster in children: findings from a pilot study.

Elder, G. H., J. K. Liker, and L. E. Cross. 1984. Parent-child behavior in the Great Depression: life course and intergenerational influences. In P. B. Baltes and O. G. Brim, Jr., eds., *Life span development and behavior,* vol. 6. New York: Academic Press.

Emery, R. E., and R. D. O'Leary. 1982. Children's perceptions of marital discord and behavior problems in boys and girls. *Journal of Abnormal Child Psychology* 10:11–24.

Garrison, W., and F. Earls. 1983. Life events and social supports in families with a two-year-old: methods and preliminary findings. *Comprehensive Psychiatry* 24:439–452.

Herjanic, B. M. 1984. Systematic diagnostic interviewing of children: present state and future possibilities. *Psychiatric Developments* 2:115–130.

Kellam, S. G., J. D. Branch, K. C. Agrawal, et al. 1975. *Mental health and going to school: the Woodlawn Program of Assessment, early intervention and evaluation.* Chicago: University of Chicago Press.

———— C. H. Brown, B. R. Rubin, et al. 1983. Paths leading to teenage psychiatric symptoms and substance abuse: developmental epidemiological studies in Woodlawn. In S. B. Guze, F. J. Earls, and J. E. Barrett, eds., *Child psychopathology and development.* New York: Raven Press.

Lewis, M., C. Feiring, C. McGuffog, et al. 1984. Predicting psychopathology in six year olds from early social relations. *Child Development* 55:123–136.

Macfarlane, J. 1938. Studies in child guidance: 1. Methodology of data collection and organization. *Monographs of the Society for Research in Child Development* 3 (serial no. 6).

Milgram, N. A. 1979. Psychological stress and adjustment in times of peace and war. *Israel Journal of Psychiatry* 40:287–291.

Quinton, D., and M. Rutter. 1984. Parents with children in care: II. Intergenerational continuities. *Journal of Child Psychology and Psychiatry* 25:231–250.

Reich, W., B. Herjanic, Z. Welner, et al. 1982. Development of a structured psychiatric interview for children: agreement on diagnosis comparing child and parent interviews. *Journal of Abnormal Child Psychology* 10:325–326.

Richman, N., J. Stevenson, and P. J. Graham. 1982. *Pre-school to school: a behavioural study.* London: Academic Press.

Rutter, M., P. Graham, O. Chadwick, et al. 1976. Adolescent turmoil: fact or fiction? *Journal of Child Psychology and Psychiatry* 17:35–56.

Rutter, M., J. Tizard, and K. Whitmore. 1970. *Education, health and behaviour.* London: Longman.

Thomas, A., and S. Chess. 1984. Genesis and evolution of behavioral disorders: from infancy to early adult life. *American Journal of Psychiatry* 141:1–9.

Wallerstein, J. S., and J. B. Kelly. 1975. The effects of parental divorce: experiences of the preschool child. *Journal of the American Academy of Child Psychiatry* 14:600–616.

Werner, E., J. Bierman, and F. French. 1971. *The children of Kauai.* Honolulu: University of Hawaii Press.

Werner, E., and R. Smith. 1979. An epidemiologic perspective on some antecedents and consequences of childhood mental health problems and learning disabilities. *Journal of the American Academy of Child Psychiatry* 18:292–306.

Yamamoto, K. 1979. Children's ratings of the stressfulness of experiences. *Developmental Psychology* 15:581–582.

3. Stress on and in the Family

Author's note: Preparation of this chapter was supported in part by a grant from the John D. and Catherine T. MacArthur Foundation.

Bowlby, J. 1973. *Separation: anxiety and anger* (vol. 2 of *Attachment and loss*). New York: Basic Books.

——— 1980. *Loss: sadness and depression* (vol. 3 of *Attachment and loss*). New York: Basic Books.

Kagan, J., J. S. Reznick, C. Clarke, N. Snidman, and C. Garcia-Coll. 1984. Behavioral inhibition to the unfamiliar. *Child Development* 55:2212–25.

Maccoby, E. E., M. E. Snow, and C. N. Jacklin. 1984. Children's dispositions and mother-child interaction at twelve and eighteen months: a short-term longitudinal study. *Developmental Psychology* 20:459–472.

4. Fathers

Bailyn, L. 1974. Accommodations as career strategy: implications for the realm of work. Working paper 728–774, Sloan School of Management, Massachusetts Institute of Technology.

Belsky, J. 1981. Early human experience: a family perspective. *Developmental Psychology* 17:3–23.

Brown, J. V., and R. Bakeman. 1980. Relationships of human mothers with their infants during the first year of life: effects of prematurity. In R. W. Bell and W. P. Smotherman, eds., *Maternal influences and early behavior.* Holliswood: Spectrum.

Cochran, M. M., and J. A. Brassard. 1979. Child development and personal social networks. *Child Development* 50:601–616.

Clarke-Stewart, K. A. 1978. Popular primers for parents. *American Psychologist* 33:359–369.

Colman, A. D., and L. L. Colman. 1971. *Pregnancy: the psychological experience.* New York: Herder.

Conway, E., and Y. Brackbill. 1970. Delivery medication and infant outcome: an empirical study. *Monographs of the Society for Research in Child Development* 35:24–34.

Dickie, J. R., and P. Matheson. 1984. Mother-father-infant: who needs support? Paper at the American Psychological Association, Toronto.

Durrett, M. E., M. Otaki, and P. Richards. 1984. Attachment and the mother's perception of support from the father. *International Journal of Behavioral Development* 7:167–176.

Emory, R. E. 1982. Interparental conflict and the children of discord and divorce. *Psychological Bulletin* 92:310–330.

Entwisle, D. R., and S. G. Doering. 1980. *The first birth.* Baltimore: Johns Hopkins University Press.

Feldman, S. S., S. C. Nash, and B. G. Aschenbrenner. 1983. Antecedents of fathering. *Child Development* 54:1628–36.

Goldberg, S., and V. DeVitto. (1983). *Born too soon.* San Francisco: Freeman.

Goldberg, W. A. 1982. Marital quality and child-mother, child-father attachments. *Infant Behavior and Development* 5:96.

Grossman, F. K., L. S. Eichler, and S. A. Winickoff. 1980 *Pregnancy, birth, and parenthood.* San Francisco: Jossey-Bass.

Henneborn, W. J., and R. Cogan. 1975. The effect of husband participation in reported pain and the probability of medication during labor and birth. *Journal of Psychosomatic Research* 19:215–222.

Hock, E. 1978. Working and nonworking mothers with infants: perceptions of their careers, their infant's needs, and satisfaction with mothering. *Developmental Psychology* 14:37–43.

——— 1980. Working and nonworking mothers and their infants: a comparative study of maternal caregiving characteristics and infant social behavior. *Merrill-Palmer Quarterly* 26:79–101.

Hoffman, L. W. 1983. Increasing fathering: effects on the mother. In M. E. Lamb and A. Sagi, eds., *Fatherhood and family policy.* Hillsdale: Erlbaum.

——— 1984. Work, family, and the socialization of the child. In R. D. Parke, R. Emde, H. McAdoo, and G. P. Sackett, eds., *Review of child development research*, vol. 7. Chicago: University of Chicago Press.

Lamb, M. E. 1977. Father-infant and mother-infant interaction in the first year of life. *Child Development* 48:167–181.

——— J. H. Pleck, and J. A. Levine. 1984. The role of the father in child development: the effects of increased paternal involvement. In B. B. Lahey and A. E. Kazdin, eds. *Advances in clinical child psychology*, vol 8. New York: Plenum.

Leifer, M. 1977. Psychological changes accompanying pregnancy and motherhood. *Genetic Psychology Monographs* 95:55–96.

Lerner, R., and G. Spanier. 1978. *Child influences on marital quality: a life-span perspective.* New York: Academic Press.

Marton, P., K. Minde, and M. Perrotta. 1981. The role of the father for the infant at risk. *American Journal of Orthopsychiatry* 51:672–679.

Murray, A. D., R. M. Dolby, R. L. Nation, and D. B. Thomas. 1981. Effects of epidural anesthesia on newborns and their mothers. *Child Development* 52:71–82.

Parke, R. D., and S. E. O'Leary. 1976. Father-mother-infant interaction in the newborn period: some findings, some observations and some unresolved issues. In K. Riegel and J. Meacham, eds., *The developing individual in a changing world,* vol. 2, *Social and environmental issues.* The Hague: Mouton.

—— and D. B. Sawin. 1976. The father's role in infancy: a re-evaluation. *Family Coordinator* 25:365–371.

—— and D. B. Sawin, 1980. The family in early infancy: social, interactional and attitudinal analyses. In F. A. Pedersen, ed., *The father-infant relationship: observational studies in the family setting.* New York: Praeger Special Studies.

—— and B. R. Tinsley. 1981. The father's role in infancy: determinants of involvement in caregiving and play. In M. E. Lamb, ed., *The role of the father in child development.* New York: Wiley.

—— and B. R. Tinsley. 1984. Fatherhood: historical and contemporary perspectives. In K. McCluskey and H. Reese, eds., *Life span development: historical and generational effects.* New York: Academic Press.

Pedersen, F. A. 1975. Mother, father, and infant as an interactive system. Paper at the American Psychological Association, Chicago.

—— ed. 1980. *The father-infant relationship: observational studies in the family setting.* New York: Praeger Special Studies.

—— R. Cain, M. Zaslow, and B. Anderson. 1980. Variation in infant experience with alternative family organization. Paper at the International Conference on Infant Studies, New Haven.

Peterson, G. H., L. E. Mehl, and P. H. Leiderman. 1979. The role of some birth-related variables in father attachment. *American Journal of Orthopsychiatry* 49:330–338.

Pleck, J. H. 1983. Husbands' paid work and family roles: current research issues. In H. Z. Lopata and J. H. Pleck, eds., *Research on the interweave of social roles,* vol. 3, *Families and jobs.* Greenwich: JAI Press.

Power, T. G., and R. D. Parke. 1984. Social network factors and the transition to parenthood. *Sex Roles* 10:949–972.

Raush, H., W. Barry, R. Hertel, and M. Swain. 1974. *Communication, conflict and marriage.* San Francisco: Jossey-Bass.

Robinson, J. P. 1977. *How Americans use time.* New York: Praeger.

Russell, G. 1982. *The changing role of fathers.* St. Lucia: University of Queensland Press.

—— and N. Radin. 1983. Increased paternal participation: the fathers' perspective. In M. E. Lamb and A. Sagi, eds., *Fatherhood and family policy.* Hillsdale: Erlbaum.

Switzky, L. T., P. Vietze, and H. Switzky. 1979. Attitudinal and demographic predictors of breast-feeding and bottle-feeding behavior in mothers of six-week-old infants. *Psychological Reports* 45:3–14.

Shereshefsky, P. M., and L. J. Yarrow. 1973. *Psychological aspects of a first pregnancy and early postnatal adaptation.* New York: Raven.

Tinsley, B. R., and R. D. Parke, 1984. Grandparents as support and socialization agents. In M. Lewis, ed., *Beyond the dyad.* New York: Plenum.

Vietze, P. M., R. H. MacTurk, M. E. McCarthy, R. P. Klein, and L. J. Yarrow. 1980. Impact of mode of delivery on father- and mother-infant interaction at 6 and 12 months. Paper at the International Conference on Infant Studies, New Haven.

Vincent, J. P. 1981. Couples and their first children: possible early signs of problems? Paper at the American Psychological Association, Los Angeles.

Walker, K. E. 1970. Time spent by husbands in household work. *Family Economics Review* 4:8–11.

———— and M. Woods. 1976. *Time use: a measure of household production of family goods and services.* Washington, D.C.: American Home Economics Association.

Yogman, M. W. 1983. Development of the father-infant relationship. In H. Fitzgerald, B. Lester, and M. W. Yogman, eds., *Theory and research in behavioral pediatrics,* vol. 1. New York: Plenum.

5. Single Mothers and Joint Custody

Anthony, E. J., and T. Benedek. 1970. *Parenthood, its psychology and psychopathology.* Boston: Little Brown.

Atkins, R. N. 1981. Finding one's father: the mother's contribution to early father representations. *Journal of the American Academy of Psychoanalysis* 9:539–559.

———— 1982. Discovering daddy: the mother's role. In S. Cath, A. Gurwitt, and J. M. Ross, eds., *Father and child.* Boston: Little Brown.

———— 1984a. Transitive vitalization and its impact on father representation. *Contemporary Psychoanalysis* 20:663–676.

———— 1984b. Joint custody: the human dilemma. Submitted for publication.

Bach, G. R. 1946. Father fantasies and father-typing in father-separated children. *Child Development* 17:63–80.

Benedek, E. P., and R. S. Benedek. 1979. Joint custody: solution or illusion? *American Journal of Psychiatry* 136:1540–44.

Benedek, T. 1959. Parenthood as a developmental phase. *Journal of the American Psychoanalytic Association* 7:389–417.

———— 1973. *Psychoanalytic investigations.* New York: Quadrangle.

Bernstein, N. R., and J. S. Robey. 1962. The detection and management of pediatric difficulties created by divorce. *Pediatrics* 45: 950–956.

Brown, S. W., and T. Harris. 1978. *The social origins of depression.* New York: Free Press.

Children's Defense Fund. 1982. *America's children and their families: key facts.* Washington, D.C.: CDF.

Derdeyn, A. 1983. The family in divorce: issues of parental anger. *Journal of the American Academy of Child Psychiatry* 22:385–391.

—— and E. Scott. 1984. Joint custody: a critical analysis and appraisal. *American Journal of Orthopsychiatry* 54:199–209.

Freud, A., and D. Burlingham. 1943. *Infants without families.* New York: International Universities Press.

Greif, J. 1979. Fathers, children, and joint custody. *American Journal of Orthopsychiatry* 49:411–419.

Hacker, A. 1983. *U/S, a statistical portrait of the american people.* New York: Viking.

Hetherington, E. M. 1979. Divorce: a child's perspective. *American Psychologist* 34:851–858.

Hilgard, J., and F. Fisk. 1960. Strength of the adult ego following childhood bereavement. *American Journal of Orthopsychiatry* 30:788–798.

Kessler, R. C. 1979. A strategy for studying the differential vulnerability to the psychological consequences of stress. *Journal of Health and Social Behavior* 20:100–108.

Leahey, M. 1984. Findings from research on divorce: implications for professionals' skill development. *American Journal of Orthopsychiatry* 298–317.

McClanahan, S. 1983. Family structure and stress: a longitudinal comparison of two-parent and female-headed households. *Journal of Marriage and the Family* 45:347–357.

Neubauer, P. 1960. The one-parent child and his oedipal development. *The Psychoanalytic Study of the Child* 15:286–309.

Olsen, T. 1956. I stand here ironing. In T. Olsen, *Tell Me a Riddle.* New York: Delacorte.

Paley, G. 1978. Faith in a tree. In S. Spinner, ed., *Motherlove, stories about motherhood.* New York: Laurel.

Parke, R. 1979. Perspectives on father-infant interaction. In J. D. Osofsky, ed., *Handbook of infant development.* New York: Wiley.

Pearlin, L. I., and J. S. Johnson. 1977. Marital status, life-stress, and depression. *American Sociological Review* 42:704–715.

Pearlin, L. I., and C. Schooler. 1978. The structure of coping. *Journal of Health and Social Behavior* 19:166–177.

Roman, M., and W. Haddad. 1978. *The disposable parent: the case for joint custody.* New York: Holt.

Rutter, M. 1971. Parent-child separation: psychological effects on the children. *Journal of Child Psychology and Psychiatry* 12:233–260.

Steinman, S. 1981. The experience of children in a joint custody arrangement: a report of a study. *American Journal of Orthopsychiatry* 51:403–414.

Wallerstein, J., and J. Kelly. 1975. The effects of parental divorce: experiences of the preschool child. *Journal of the American Academy of Child Psychiatry* 14:600–616.

—— 1980. *Surviving the breakup: how children and parents cope with divorce.* New York: Basic Books.

Weinraub, M., and B. M. Wolf. 1983. Effects of stress and social supports on mother-child interactions in single- and two-parent families. *Child Development* 54:1297–1311.

Weiss, R. 1979. *Going it alone: the family life and social situation of the single parent.* New York: Basic Books.

Yogman, M., R. D. Parke, R. N. Atkins, and J. Pleck. 1984. Current issues in fatherhood research, panel discussion at the biannual meeting of the ICIS, April 1984.

6. Working It Out

Belsky, J. 1981. Early human experience: a family perspective. *Developmental Psychology* 17.3–23.

Berscheid, E., and L. A. Peplau. 1983. The emerging science of relationships. In H. Kelley et al., *Close relationships.* New York: Freeman.

Blood, R. O., Jr., and D. M. Wolfe. 1960. *Husbands and wives.* New York: Free Press.

Bronfenbrenner, U., and A. C. Crouter. 1982. Work and family through time and space. In S. Kamerman and C. Hayes, eds., *Families that work: children in a changing world.* Washington, D.C.: National academy of Sciences.

—— W. F. Alvarez, and C. R. Henderson, Jr. 1984. Working and watching: maternal employment status and parents' perceptions of their three-year-old children. *Child Development* 55(4):1362–78.

Burke, R. J., and T. Weir. 1981. Impact of occupational demands on nonwork experiences. *Group and Organization Studies* 6(4):472–485.

Crouter, A. C. 1984a. Participative work as an influence on human development. *Journal of Applied Developmental Psychology* 5(1):71–90.

—— 1984b. Spillover from family to work: the neglected side of the work-family interface. *Human Relations* 37:425–442.

——M. Perry-Jenkins, and T. L. Huston. In preparation. The spillover of moods generated at work to family relationships and activities.

Elder, G. H., Jr. 1974. *Children of the great depression.* Chicago: University of Chicago Press.

Gianopulos, A., and H. E. Mitchell. 1957. Marital disagreement in working wife marriages as a function of husband's attitude toward wife's employment. *Marriage and Family Living* 19:373–378.

Goldberg, S. 1977. Social competence in infancy: a model of parent-infant interaction. *Merrill-Palmer Quarterly* 23:163–177.

Heath, D. B. 1977. Some possible effects of occupation on the maturing of professional men. *Journal of Vocational Behavior* 11:263–281.

Huston, T. L. 1983. Power. In H. Kelley et al., *Close relationships.* New York: Freeman.

—— S. M. McHale, and A. C. Crouter. In press. When the honeymoon's over: changes in the marriage relationship over the first year. In R. Gilmour and S. Duck, eds., *The emerging field of personal relationships.* Hillsdale: Erlbaum.

Kanter, R. M. 1977. *Work and family in the United States: a critical review and agenda for research and policy.* New York: Russell Sage Foundation.

Kohn, M. L. 1969. *Class and conformity: a study in values.* Homewood: Dorsey Press.

Komarovsky, M. 1940. *The unemployed man and his family.* New York: Dryden Press.

Locke, H. J., and M. Mackeprang, M. 1949. Marital adjustment and the employed wife. *American Journal of Sociology* 54:536–538.

McHale, S. M., and T. L. Huston. 1984. Men and women as parents: sex role orientations, employment, and parental roles with infants. *Child Development* 55(4):1349–61.

Mott, P. E., F. C. Mann, Q. McLoughlin, and D. P. Warwick. 1965. *Shift work: the social, psychological, and physical consequences.* Ann Arbor: University of Michigan Press.

Nye, I. 1959. Employment status of mothers and marital conflict, permanence, and happiness. *Social Problems* 6:260–267.

Pleck, J. H. 1983. Husbands' paid work and family roles: current research issues. In H. Lopata and J. H. Pleck, eds., *Research in the interweave of social roles, vol. 3: Families and jobs.* Greenwich: JAI Press.

Rapoport, R., and R. N. Rapoport. 1976. *Dual-career families re-examined.* London: Martin Robertson; New York: Harper and Row.

Rivers, C., R. Barnett, and G. Baruch. 1979. *Beyond sugar and spice.* New York: Putnam's.

Rockwell, R. C., and G. H. Elder. 1982. Economic deprivation and problem behavior: childhood and adolescence in the great depression. *Human Development* 25:57–64.

Smelser, N. J. 1980. Issues in the study of work and love in adulthood. In N. J. Smelser and E. H. Erikson, eds., *Themes of work and love in adulthood.* Cambridge: Harvard University Press.

Voydanoff, P. 1980. *The implications of work-family relationships for productivity.* Scarsdale: Work in America Institute.

———— 1983. Unemployment: family strategies for adaptation. In C. R. Figley and H. I. McCubbin, eds., *Stress and the family, vol. 2: Catastrophic stressors.* New York: Brunner Mazel.

Walker, K., and M. Woods. 1976. *Time use: a measure of household production of family goods and services.* Washington: Home Economics Association.

Waller, W. W. 1938. *The family: a dynamic interpretation.* New York: Cordan.

Weatherly, U. G. (1909). How does the access of women to industrial occupations react on the family? *American Journal of Sociology* 14:740–765.

7. Family Life and Corporate Policies

Author's note: I am indebted to the following colleagues for reading and commenting on this chapter: Karen Blum, Richard Ruopp, Judy David, Peggy Simpson McGinley, Diane Hughes, Arthur F. Strohmer, Susan Jenkins, Marjorie Acosta, Sheila Kamerman, Susan Ginsberg, and Dana Friedman.

Axel, H. 1985. *Corporations and families: changing practices and perspectives.* New York: The Conference Board.

Barnett, R. G. and G. K. Baruch. 1983. Women's involvement in multiple roles, role strain, and psychological stress. Wellesley: Wellesley College Center for Research on Women.

Belle, D. 1982. *Social support, lives in stress: women in depression.* Beverly Hills: Sage.

Belsky, J., M. Perry-Jenkins, and A. C. Crouter. 1985. The work-family interface and marital change across the transition to parenthood. *Journal of Family Issues* 6(2):205–220.

—— L. D. Steinberg, and A. Walker. 1982. The ecology of daycare: parenting and child development. In M. E. Lamb, ed., *Nontraditional families.* Hillsdale: Erlbaum.

Blank, H. April 1984. Testimony of the Children's Defense Fund before the Joint Economic Committee concerning child-care problems faced by working mothers and pregnant women. Washington, D.C.

Bohen, H. H. 1983. *Employment policies affecting families and children: the United States and Europe.* New York: Aspen Institute for Humanistic Studies.

—— and A. Viveros-Long. 1981. *Balancing job and family life.* Philadelphia: Temple University Press.

Bronfenbrenner, U., and A. C. Crouter. 1982. Work and family through time and space. In S. R. Kamerman and C. D. Hayes, eds., *Families that work: children in a changing world.* Washington, D.C.: National Academy Press.

Bureau of Labor Statistics, U.S. Department of Labor. 1982. *Employee benefits in medium and large firms.* Washington, D.C.: Government Printing Office.

—— 1984. *Current population survey* (March supplement). Washington, D.C.: Government Printing Office.

Burud, S. L., P. R. Aschbacher, and J. McCroskey. 1984. *Employer-supported child care.* Boston: Auburn House.

Carlson, B. E. 1984. The father's contribution to child care: effects on children's perception of parental roles. *American Journal of Orthopsychiatry* 54:123–136.

Catalyst. 1981. *Corporations and two-career families.* New York: Author.

——1983. *Corporate relocation practices: A report on a nationwide survey.* New York: Author.

——1984. *Work and family seminars: corporations' response to employees' needs.* New York: Author.

Children's Defense Fund. 1982. *Employed parents and their children: a data book.* Washington, D.C.: Author.

—— 1984. *A children's defense budget.* Washington, D.C.: Author.

Cobb, S. 1979. Social support as a moderation of life stress. *Psychosomatic Medium* 38(5):300–314.

Collins, G. July 9, 1984. Lawyers share jobs for more family time. *New York Times,* p. B6.

Crouter, A. C. 1984. Spillover from family to work: the neglected side of work-family interface. *Human Relations* 37(6):425–442.

De la Mare, G., and S. Walker. 1968. Factors influencing the choice of shift rotation. *Occupational Psychology* 42:1–21.

Emlen, A. C. and P. E. Koren. 1984. *Hard to find and difficult to manage: the effects of child care on the workplace.* Portland: Regional Institute for Human Services.

Fernandez, J. 1985. Child care and corporate productivity: resolving family/ work conflict. New York: Lexington Books, D.C. Heath

Friedman, D. E. 1983. *Encouraging employer support to working parents.* New York: Carnegie Corporation.

———— May 1984. Speech at Swedish Information Service Conference. New York.

———— 1985. Corporate financial assistance for child care. *Conference Board Research Bulletin* 177. New York: The Conference Board.

Galinsky, E., and W. H. Hooks, 1977. *The new extended family: day care that works.* Boston: Houghton Mifflin.

———— R. R. Ruopp, and K. S. Blum. 1983. Work and family life study. Unpublished data.

Gottlieb, B. H. 1978. The development and application of a classification scheme of informal helping behaviors. *Canadian Journal of Behavioral Science* 10:105–115.

Grossman, A. S. 1979. *Employment in perspective: working women* (Report 565). Washington, D.C.: Bureau of Labor Statistics, U.S. Department of Labor.

Haldi Associates. 1977. Summary report of findings of a comprehensive psychology assessment of alternative work schedules. New York: Author.

Lou Harris and Associates, Inc. 1981. Families at work: strengths and strains. The General Mills American Family Forum. Minneapolis: General Mills.

Heath, D. B. 1977. Some possible effects of occupation on the maturing of professional men. *Journal of Vocational Behavior* 11:263–281.

Hewlitt, S. A. 1983. Parents and work: family policy in comparative perspective. Proposal by the Economic Policy Council (UNA-USA).

Hock, E. 1979. Working and nonworking mothers and their infants: a comparative study of maternal caregiving characteristics and infant social behavior. Columbus: Ohio State University (mimeo).

House, J. S. 1981. *Work stress and social support.* Reading: Addison-Wesley.

Hughes, D. 1985. Work-family interference. Unpublished manuscript.

Hunt, J. G., and L. L. Hunt. 1977. Dilemmas and contradictions of status: the case of the dual career family. *Social Problems* 24:407–416.

Kamerman, S. B. 1983. *Meeting family needs: the corporate response.* Work in America Institute Studies in Productivity. New York: Pergamon.

———— and A. J. Kahn. 1981. *Child care, family benefits, and working parents.* New York: Columbia University Press.

————and P. W. Kingston, 1982. Employer responses to the family responsibilities of employees. In S. B. Kamerman and C. D. Hayes, eds., *Families that work: children in a changing world.* Washington, D.C.: National Academy Press.

———— A. J. Kahn, and P. W. Kingston. 1983. *Maternity policies and working women.* New York: Columbia University Press.

Kanter, R. M. (1977). *Work and family in the United States: a critical review and agenda for research and policy.* New York: Russell Sage Foundation.

Keith, P. M., and R. B. Schafer. 1980. Role strain and depression in two-job families. *Family Relations* 29:483–488.

Keller Brown, L., and J. Kagan. May 1982. The working women survey: a survey of where corporate women are now and what they want next. *Working Woman* 7(5):92–96.

Kiez, A., and V. Cohen. 1979. *American Management Associations survey report of executive stress.* New York: AMACOM.

Kirk, R. J. 1981. *Alternative work schedules experimental program: interim report to the president and the congress.* Washington, D.C.: U.S. Office of Personnel Management, Office of Compensation Program Development.

Lazarus, R. S., and R. Launier. 1978. Stress-related transactions between person and environment. In L. A. Pervin and M. Lewis, eds., *Perspectives in International Psychology.* New York: Plenum.

Leavitt, R. 1983. *Employee assistance and counseling programs.* New York: Community Council of Greater New York.

Lein, L., M. Durham, M. Pratt, M. Schudson, R. Thomas, and H. Weiss. 1974. Final report: work and family life. Wellesley: Wellesley College Center for Research on Women.

Levinson, D. J., C. N. Darrow, E. B. Klein, M. H. Levinson, and B. McKee. 1978. *The seasons of a man's life.* New York: Knopf.

Levinson, H., A. G. Spohn, and J. Molinari. 1972. *Organizational diagnosis.* Cambridge: Harvard University Press.

Lodahl, T. M., and M. Kejner. 1965. The definition of job involvement. *Journal of Applied Psychology* 49(1):24–33.

Magid, R. Y. 1983. *Child care initiatives for working parents: why employees get involved.* New York: American Management Associations.

Mason, T., and R. Espinoza. 1983. Executive summary of the final report: working parents project, Washington, D.C.: National Institute of Education.

Meier, G. S. 1979. Job sharing: a new pattern for quality of work and life. Kalamazoo: W.E. Upjohn Institute for Employment Research.

Milkovich, G. T., and L. R. Gomez. 1976. Daycare and selected employee work behaviors. *Academy of Management Journal* 19(1):1111–115.

Miller, T. I. 1984. The effects of employer-sponsored child care on employee absenteeism, turnover, productivity, recruitment or job satisfaction: what is claimed and what is known. *Personnel Psychology* 37:277–289.

Money. May 1985. Going for it all, pp. 108–146.

Morgan, G. G. Unpublished. Supply and demand for child day care: the need for data.

Mott, P. E., F. C. Mann, Q. McLoughlin, and D. P. Warwick. 1965. Shift work: the social, psychological, and physical consequences. Ann Arbor: University of Michigan Press.

New York State Council on Child and Families. 1983. *Part-time employment: implications for families and the workplace.*

Nollen, S. D. 1982. *New work schedules in practice: managing time in a changing society.* New York: Van Nostrand Reinhold.

Olmsted, B., and S. Smith. 1983. *The job sharing handbook.* New York: Penguin.

Ouchi, W. 1981. *Theory Z: how Americans can meet the Japanese challenge.* Reading: Addison-Wesley.

Pearlin L. I., and C. Schooler 1978. The structure of coping. *Journal of Health of Social Behavior* 19(3):2–21.

Perry, K. S. 1978. Survey and analysis of employer-sponsored day care in the U.S. Unpublished doctoral dissertation, University of Wisconsin, Milwaukee.

Peters, T. J., and R. H. Waterman, Jr. 1983. *In search of excellence.* New York: Warner.

Piotrkowski, C. S. 1979. *Work and the family system: a naturalistic study of working-class and lower-middle-class families.* New York: Free Press.

——— May 1985. Research Interest Group Presentation. New York: Bank Street College.

——— and P. Crits-Christoph. 1982. Women's jobs and family adjustment. In J. Aldous, ed., *Two paychecks: life in dual-earner families.* Beverly Hills: Sage.

Pirie, V. 1985. Balancing work and parent care responsibilities. Unpublished manuscript.

Pleck, J. H. 1977. The work-family role system. *Social Problems* 24:417–427.

——— (1979). Men's family work: three perspectives and some new data. *Family Coordinator* 28:481–88.

——— (1983). Husband's paid work and family roles: current research issue. In H. Lopata and J. H. Pleck, eds., *Research on the interview of social roles: women and men,* vol. 3. Greenwich: JAI Press.

——— Unpublished. Employment: the working father. Manuscript.

——— and Rustad 1980. Husbands and wives time in family work and paid work in the 1975–76 study of time use. Wellesley: Wellesley College Center for Research on Women.

——— and G. L. Staines. 1983. Work schedules and work family conflict in two earner couples. In J. Aldous, ed., *Dual earner families.* Beverly Hills: Sage.

———G. L. Staines, and L. Lang. 1978. Work and family life: first reports on work-family interference and workers formal child-care arrangements from the 1977 Quality of Employment Survey. Wellesley: Wellesley College Center for Research on Women.

——— G. L. Staines, and L. Lang. 1980. Conflicts between work and family. *Monthly Labor Review* 103(3):29–32.

Plewes, T. 1984. *Part-time employment in America.* McLean, Virginia: Association of Part-Time Professionals.

Quinn, R. P., and G. L. Staines. 1979. *The 1977 Quality of Employment Survey:*

descriptive statistics with comparison data from the 1969–70 and 1972–73 surveys. Ann Arbor: Institute for Social Research.

Rapoport, R., and R. Rapoport. 1971. *Dual-career families.* Baltimore: Penguin.

——— 1976. *Dual-career families re-examined.* Baltimore: Penguin.

Renshaw, J. 1976. An exploration of the dynamics of the overlapping worlds of work and family. *Family Process* 15(1):143–165.

Robinson, J. P. 1977. *How Americans use time: a social-psychological analysis.* New York: Praeger.

———P. E. Converse, and A. Szalai. 1972. Everyday life in twelve countries. In A. Szalai et al., eds., *The use of time.* The Hague: Mouton.

Runzheimer and Company. 1979. *A study of relocation policies among major corporations.* White Plains: Merrill Lynch Relocation Management.

Ruopp, R. R., and J. Travers. 1982. Janus faces day care: perspectives on quality and cost. In E. F. Zigler and E. W. Gordon, eds., *Daycare: scientific and social policy issues.* Boston: Auburn.

Russell, G. 1982. Shared caregiving families: an Australian study. In M. E. Lamb, ed., *Non-traditional families: parenting and child development.* Hillsdale: Erlbaum.

Saleh, D., and J. Hosak. 1976. Job involvement concepts and measurements. *Academy of Management Journal* 19:213–224.

Schmidt, W. H., and B. Z. Posner. 1983. *Managerial values in perspective.* New York: American Management Associations.

Seligson, M., A. Genser, E. Gannett, and W. Gray. 1983. *School-age child care: a policy report.* Wellesley: School-Age Child Care Project.

Shinn, M., M. Rosario, H. Mørch, and D. E. Chestnut. In press. Job stress and burnout. *Journal of Personality.*

Silverman, P. May 1984. Speech at the Family Resource Coalition Conference, New York.

Simon, J., and W. Mares. 1982. *Working together.* New York: Knopf.

Skinner, D. A., and H. I. McCubbin, 1982. Coping in dual-employed families: spousal differences. Mimeo.

Slocum, W. L., and F. I. Nye. 1976. Provider and housekeeper roles. In F. I. Nye et al., eds., *Role structure and analysis of the family.* Beverly Hills: Russell Sage Foundation.

Smith, R. E., ed. 1979. *The subtle revolution.* Washington, D.C.: The Urban Institute.

Staines, G. L., and J. H. Pleck, 1983. *The impact of work schedules on the family.* Ann Arbor: Institute for Social Research.

Toffler, A. 1980. *The third wave.* New York: Morrow.

Unger, D., and D. Powell. 1980. Supporting families under stress: the role of social networks. *Family Relations* 29:566–574.

U.S. Bureau of the Census. 1983. Child care arrangements of working mothers: June 1982, series P.23, no. 129. Washington D.C.: Government Printing Office.

U.S. Department of Labor, Women's Bureau. 1983. Employers and child care: establishing services through the workplace. Washington D.C.: Department of Labor.

Winett, R. A., and M. S. Neale. 1981. Flexible work schedules and family time allocation: assessment of a system change on individual behavior using self-report logs. *Journal of Applied Behavior Analysis* 1:41–51.

——— M. E. Neale, and K. Williams. 1982. The Effect of flexible work schedules on urban families with young children: quasi-experimental ecology studies. *American Journal of Community Psychology* 10:29–64.

Yarrow, M. R., P. Scott, L. DeLeeuw, and C. Meining. 1962. Childrearing in families of working and non-working mothers. *Sociometry* 25:122–140.

Yogev S., and S. Brett. 1983. Patterns of work and family involvement among single and dual earner couples: two competing analytical approaches. Washington D.C.: Office of Naval Research.

8. Utilitarianism

Freud, S. 1911. Psychoanalytic notes upon an autobiographical account of a case of paranoia. Reprinted in *Three Case Histories*. New York: Crowell-Collier, 1963.

Zaleznik, A. 1977. Managers and leaders: are they different? *Harvard Business Review* 55:67–78.

——— 1979. Isolation and control in the family and work. In T. B. Brazelton and V. Vaughan, eds., *The family: setting priorities*. New York: Science and Medicine.

9. Supplemental Care for Young Children

Aronson, S. June 1984. Paper at Conference on Infectious Disease, Minneapolis.

Clarke-Stewart, A. 1978. *Child care in the family*. New York: Academic Press.

Fein, G. 1979. Infant day care and the family: regulatory strategies to ensure parent participation. Prepared for Assistant Secretary for Planning and Evaluation, DHHS. Detroit: Merrill-Palmer Institute.

Hofferth, S. L. 1979. Day care in the next decade, 1980–1990. *Journal of Marriage and the Family* 41(3):649–658.

Johnson, L., et al. 1980. *Comparative licensing study*. Washington, D.C.: Prepared for DHHS, Administration for Children, Youth and Families, updated 1982.

Kamerman, S. 1983. The child care debate: working mothers vs. America. *Working Woman* November.

Kennedy, E. 1982. Child care—a commitment to be honored. In E. Zigler and E. Gordon, eds., *Day care: scientific and social policy issues*. Boston: Auburn House.

Lazar, I. September 1977. *The persistence of preschool effects*. Washington, D.C.: Report by central staff of Consortium for Longitudinal Studies; DHEW OHDS, final report to administration for Children, Youth and Families.

Levine, J. 1982. The prospects and dilemmas of child care information and referral. In E. Zigler and E. Gordon, eds., *Day care: scientific and social policy issues*. Boston: Auburn House.

Mohlabane, N. 1984. Infants in day care centers, "in sickness and in health." Master's thesis, Pacific Oaks college. Oakland: Bananas.

Moore, J. 1980. *Parent decisions on the use of day care and early education services: an analysis of amount used and type chosen*. Ann Arbor: University Microfilms.

Morgan, G. 1982. Demystifying the day care delivery system. Paper at Wheelock College Conference on Delivery Systems, Boston.

——— 1984. Change through regulation. In R. Fuqua and J. Greenman, eds., *Making day care better*. New York: Columbia University Teachers' College Press.

Parents in the Workplace. July 1983. *Sick child care, a problem for working parents and employers*. Minneapolis.

Preschool Association of the West Side. 1980. Working draft. New York: Bank Street College of Education.

Project Connections. 1978–1982. Final report. Unpublished study of information and referral services for Administration for Children, Youth and Families and the Ford Foundation, by American Institutes for Research, Cambridge, Mass.

Rhodes, T. W., and J. C. Moore. 1976. *National child care consumer study, 1975*. Washington, D.C.: DHEW Office of Child Development.

Prescott, E., and T. David. 1978. Concept paper on the effects of the physical environment on day care. Pasadena: Pacific Oaks College.

——— E. Jones, et al. 1967, 1972. *Group day care as a child-rearing environment: an observational study of day care programs*. Pasadena: Pacific Oaks College. Vol. 2 (1972), Washington, D.C.: National Association for the Education of Young Children.

Richmond, J., and J. Janis. 1982. Health care services for children in day care programs. In E. Zigler and E. Gordon, eds., *Day care: scientific and social policy issues*. Boston: Auburn House.

Ruopp, R., et al. 1973. *A day care guide for administrators, teachers, and parents*. Cambridge: MIT Press.

——— J. Travers, F. Glantz, and C. Coelen. 1979. *Children at the center*. Cambridge: Abt Associates.

Shipman, V. 1976. *Disadvantaged children and their first school experience*. Princeton: Educational Testing Service.

U.S. Census Bureau. 1976. *Daytime care of children, October 1974 and February 1975*. Washington, D.C.: Government Printing Office.

——— 1982. *Trends in child care arrangements of working mothers*. Washington, D.C.: Government Printing Office.

Vogt, L., et al. 1973. *Health start: final report of the evaluation of the second year program*. Washington, D.C.: Urban Institute.

Weiner, S. 1978. The child care market in Seattle and Denver. In P. K. Robins and S. Weiner, *Child care and public policy*. Lexington: Lexington Books.

Whitbread, J. 1977. Family Circle child care survey. *Family Circle* February.

10. Family Adaptation to Divorce

Author's note: My sincere appreciation to colleagues and friends who provided me with helpful suggestions in preparing this chapter: Nancy Rambusch, Gary Resnik, and Donald Wertlieb.

Ahrons, C. R. 1980. Redefining the divorced family: a conceptual framework. *Social Work* 25(6):437–441.

———1981. The continuing coparental relationship between divorced spouses. *American Journal of Orthopsychiatry* 51:3.

Baker, O. V., J. Druckman, J. Flagle, K. A. Camara, C. Dayton, J. Egan, and A. Cohen, A. 1980. *The identification and development of community-based approaches for meeting the social and emotional needs of youth and families in variant family configurations: final report.* Palo Alto: American Institutes for Research.

Barnard, J. 1972. *The future of marriage.* New York: Bantam.

Bloom, B. L., S. J. Asher, and S. W. White. 1978. Marital disruption as a stressor: a review and analysis. *Psychological Bulletin* 85:867–894.

———W. F. Hodges, and R. A. Caldwell. 1982. A preventive intervention program for the newly separated: initial evaluation. *American Journal of Community Psychology* 10:251–264.

Bohannan, P., ed. 1971. *Divorce and after.* New York: Anchor.

Brown, P. 1976. Psychological distress and personal growth among women coping with marital dissolution. Dissertation, University of Michigan.

Burr, W. F. 1973. *Theory construction and the sociology of the family.* New York: Wiley.

Caldwell, R. A., and B. L. Bloom. 1982 Social support: its structure and impact on marital disruption. *American Journal of Community Psychology* 10(6):647–667.

Camara, K. A. 1979. Children's construction of social knowledge: concepts of family and the experience of parental divorce. Dissertation, Stanford University.

——— 1985. For the sake of the children: interparental cooperation and conflict after divorce. Paper at the American Orthopsychiatric Association Annual Conference, New York.

———O. V. Baker, and C. Dayton. 1980. Impact of separation and divorce on youths and families. In P. M. Insel, ed., *Environmental variables and the prevention of mental illness.* Lexington: D. C. Heath.

Cherlin, A. 1981. *Marriage, divorce, remarriage.* Cambridge: Harvard University Press.

Cobb, S. 1976. Social support as a moderator of life stress. *Psychosomatic Medicine* 38:300–314.

Coletta, M. D. 1979. Support systems after divorce: incidence and impact. *Journal of Marriage and the Family* 41:837–846.

Dunn, J., C. Kendrick, and R. McNamee. 1981. The reaction of first-born children to the birth of a sibling: mothers' reports. *Journal of Child Psychology and Psychiatry* 22:1–18.

George, L. 1980. *Role transitions in later life.* Belmont, Calif.: Brooks/Cole.

Hess, R. D., and K. A. Camara. 1979. Post-divorce family relationships as mediating factors in the consequences of divorce for children. *Journal of Social Issues* 35:79–96.

Hetherington, E. M. 1981. Children and divorce. In R. Henderson, ed., *Parent-child interaction: theory, research and prospect.* New York: Academic Press.

———— and K. A. Camara. 1984. Families in transition: the processes of dissolution and reconstitution. In R. Parke, ed., *Review of child development research,* vol. 7. Chicago: University of Chicago Press.

———— K. A. Camara, and D. L. Featherman. 1982. *Cognitive performance, school behavior and achievement of children from one-parent households.* Washington, D.C.: National Institute of Education.

———— M. Cox, and R. Cox. 1979. Family interaction and the social, emotional and cognitive development of children following divorce. In V. Vaughan and T. B. Brazelton, eds., *The family: setting priorities.* New York: Science and Medicine.

———— 1982. Effects of divorce on parents and children. In M. Lamb, ed., *Nontraditional families.* Hillsdale: Erlbaum.

Jacobson, D. S. 1978. The impact of divorce/separation on children. III. Parent-child communication and child adjustment: regression analysis of findings from overall study. *Journal of Divorce* 2:175–194.

Kalter, N. 1977. Children of divorce in an outpatient psychiatric population. *American Journal of Orthopsychiatry* 47:1.

———— J. Pickar, and M. Lesowitz. 1984. School-based developmental facilitation groups for children of divorce: a preventive intervention. *American Journal of Orthopsychiatry* 54:613–623.

Kelly, J. B., and J. S. Wallerstein. 1977. Brief interventions with children in divorcing families. *American Journal of Orthopsychiatry* 47:23–29.

Kitson, G. C., and H. J. Raschke. 1981. Divorce research: what we know, what we need to know. *Journal of Divorce* 4:1–37.

McCall, R. B., and S. H. Stocking. 1980. *Divorce: a summary of research about the effects of divorce on families.* Boys Town: Boys Town Center Communications and Public Service Division.

McLanahan, S. S., N. V. Wedemeyer, and T. Adelberg. 1981. Network structure, social support and psychological well-being in the single-parent family. *Journal of Marriage and the Family* 43:601–612.

Miller, A. A. 1971. Reactions of friends to divorce. In P. Bohannan, ed., *Divorce and after.* New York: Anchor.

Minuchin, P. 1985. Families and individual development: provocations from the field of family therapy. *Child Development* 56(2):289–302.

Reiss, D. 1981. *The family's construction of reality.* Cambridge: Harvard University Press.

Rutter, M. 1983. Stress, coping and development: some issues and some questions. In N. Garmezy and M. Rutter, eds., *Stress, coping and development in children.* New York: McGraw-Hill.

Santrock, J. W., and R. A. Warshak. 1979. Father custody and social development in boys and girls. *Journal of Social Issues* 35:112–125.

Shinn, M. 1978. Father absence and children's cognitive development. *Psychological Bulletin* 85:295–324.

Spicer, J., and G. Hampe. 1975. Kinship interaction after divorce. *Journal of Marriage and the Family* 28:113–119.

Wallerstein, J. S., and J. B. Kelly. 1980. *Surviving the breakup: how children and parents cope with divorce.* New York: Basic Books.

Walsh, F. 1982. Conceptualizations of normal family functioning. In F. Walsh, ed., *Normal family processes.* New York: Guilford Press.

Weiss, R. S. 1975. *Marital separation.* New York: Basic Books.

———— 1979. Growing up a little faster: the experience of growing up in a single-parent household. *Journal of Social Issues* 35:97–111.

Weitzman. L. J. 1981. The economics of divorce: social and economic consequences of property, alimony and child custody awards. *UCLA Law Review* 28:1181–1268.

Wertlieb, D. W., S. Budman, A. Demby, and M. R. Randall. 1984. Marital separation and health: stress and intervention. *Journal of Human Stress* 10:18–26.

11. The Family and Chronic Illness in Children

Author's note: Preparation of this chapter was supported in part by the W. T. Grant Foundation, the March of Dimes, and the Robert Wood Johnson Foundation.

Allan, J., R. Townley, and P. Phelan. 1974. Family response to cystic fibrosis. *Australian Paediatrics Journal* 10:136–146.

Association for the Care of Children's Health. 1984. *Home care for children with serious handicapping conditions.* Report on conference sponsored by the Association for the Care of Children's Health and the Division of Maternal and Child Health, Public Health Service, U.S. Department of Health and Human Services, Washington, D.C.

Blacher, J., ed. 1984. *Severely handicapped young children and their families.* New York: Academic Press.

Breslau, N., K. S. Staruch, and E. A. Mortimer. 1985. Psychological distress in mothers of disabled children. *American Journal of Diseases of Children* 136:682–686.

———— M. Weitzman, and K. Messenger. 1981. Psychologic functioning of siblings of disabled children. *Pediatrics* 67:344–353.

Case, J., and S. Mathews. 1983. CHIP: The Chronic Health Impaired Program of the Baltimore city public school system. *Children's Health Care* 12:97–99.

Cummings, S. T. 1976. The impact of the child's deficiencies on the father:

a study of fathers of mentally retarded and of chronically ill children. *American Journal of Orthopsychiatry* 46:246–255.

Davis, P. 1985. Personal communication.

Drotar, D., C. F. Doershuk, R. C. Stern, T. F. Boat, W. Boyer, and L. Mathews. 1981. Psychosocial functioning of children with cystic fibrosis. *Pediatrics* 67:338–343.

Featherstone, H. 1980. *A difference in the family: life with a disabled child.* New York: Basic Books.

Fowler, M. G., M. P. Johnson, and S. S. Atkinson. 1985. School achievement and absence in children with chronic health conditions. *Journal of Pediatrics* 106:683–687.

Gliedman, J., and W. Roth. 1980. *The unexpected minority: handicapped children in America: a report of the Carnegie Council on Children.* New York: Harcourt Brace Jovanovich.

Gortmaker, S. L., and W. Sappenfield. 1984. Chronic childhood disorders: prevalence and impact. *Pediatric Clinics of North America* 31:3–18.

Gross, R. H. 1985. Newborns with myelodysplasia—the rest of the story. *New England Journal of Medicine* 312:1632–34.

Haggerty, R. J., ed. 1984. Symposium on chronic disease in children. *Pediatric Clinics of North America* 31:1–277.

Heller, A., S. Rafman, I. Zvagulis, and I. B. Pless. 1985. Birth defects and psychosocial adjustment. *American Journal of Diseases of Children* 139:257–263.

Hoare, P. 1984. The development of psychiatric disorder among school children with epilepsy. *Developmental Medicine and Child Neurology* 26:3–13.

Koocher, G. R., and J. E. O'Malley. 1981. *The Damocles syndrome: psychosocial consequences of surviving childhood cancer.* New York: McGraw Hill.

Lavigne, J. V., and M. Ryan. 1979. Psychologic adjustment of siblings of children with chronic illness. *Pediatrics* 63:616–627.

Leventhal, J. M. 1984. Psychosocial assessment of children with chronic physical disease. *Pediatric Clinics of North America* 31:71–86.

——— B. F. Sabbeth, E. B. Emmons, W. Tamborlane, T. F. Dolan, and A. Berg. 1984. Do parents discuss the illness with their chronically ill child? Paper at the Ambulatory Pediatric Association, San Francisco.

Lewis, B. L., and K. T. Khaw. 1982. Family functioning as a mediating variable affecting psychosocial adjustment of children with cystic fibrosis. *Journal of Pediatrics* 101:636–640.

Liebman, R., S. Minuchin, and L. Baker. 1974. The use of structural family therapy in the treatment of intractable asthma. *American Journal of Psychiatry* 131:535–540.

MacKeith, R. 1973. The feelings and behavior of parents of handicapped children. *Developmental Medicine and Child Neurology* 15:524–527.

McAnarney, E. R., I. B. Pless, B. Satterwhite, and S. Friedman. 1974. Psychosocial problems of children with juvenile rheumatoid arthritis. *Pediatrics* 53:523–528.

McLaughlin, J. F., D. B. Shurtleff, J. Lamers, T. Stuntz, P. W. Hayden, and

R. J. Kropp. 1985. Influence of prognosis on decisions regarding the care of newborns with myelodysplasia. *New England Journal of Medicine* 312:1589–94.

Moretti, M. M., S. Fine, G. Haley, and K. Marriage. 1985. Childhood and adolescent depression: child-report versus parent-report information. *Journal of Child Psychiatry* 24:298–302.

Newacheck, P. W., P. P. Budetti, and P. McManus. 1984. Trends in childhood disability. *American Journal of Public Health* 74:232–236.

Olshansky, S. 1962. Chronic sorrow: a response to having a mentally defective child. *Social Casework* 43:190–193.

Olson, D. H., D. H. Sprenkle, and C. S. Russell. 1979. Circumplex model of marital and family systems. 1. Cohesion and adaptability dimensions, family types, and clinical application. *Family Process* 18:3–27.

Perrin, J. M., and H. T. Ireys. 1984. The organization of services for chronically ill children and their families. *Pediatric Clinics of North America* 31:235–257.

Pierce, P. M., and S. A. Freedman. 1983. The REACH project: an innovative health delivery model for medically dependent children. *Children's Health Care* 11:86–89.

Pless, I. B. 1983. Effects of chronic illness on adjustment: Clinical implications. In P. Firestone, P. J. McGrath, and W. Feldman, eds., *Advances in behavioral medicine for children and adults.* Hillsdale: Erlbaum.

——— and P. Pinkerton. 1973. *Chronic childhood disorder—promoting patterns of adjustment.* London: Henry Kimpton.

——— and R. J. Roghmann. 1971. Chronic illness and its consequences: observations based on three epidemiologic surveys. *Journal of Pediatrics* 79:351–359.

——— and B. Satterwhite. 1972. Chronic illness in childhood: selection, activities, and evaluation of non-professional family counselors. *Clinical Pediatrics* 11:403–410.

Sabbeth, B. F., J. M. Leventhal, and E. Emmons. 1984. Fathers of chronically ill children. Paper at the American Orthopsychiatric Association, Toronto.

——— and J. M. Leventhal. 1984. Marital adjustment to chronic childhood illness: a critique of the literature. *Pediatrics* 73:762–768.

Solnit, A. J., and M. H. Stark. 1961. Mourning and the birth of a defective child. *Psychoanalytic Study of the Child* 16:523–537.

Stein, R. E. K., and D. J. Jessop. 1984. Does pediatric home care make a difference for children with chronic illness? Findings from the Pediatric Ambulatory Care Treatment Study. *Pediatrics* 73:845–853.

Tew, B., and K. M. Laurence. 1973. Mothers, brothers and sisters of patients with spina bifida. *Developmental Medicine and Child Neurology* 15:69–76.

Vance, J., L. E. Fazan, B. Satterwhite, and I. B. Pless. 1980. Effects of nephrotic syndrome on the family. *Pediatrics* 65:948–956.

Walker, D. K. 1984. Care of chronically ill children in schools. *Pediatric Clinics of North America* 31:221–234.

Walker, J., M. Thomas, and I. Russel. 1971. Spina bifida—and the parents. *Developmental Medicine and Child Neurology* 13:462–476.

Weissman, M. M., H. Orvaschel, and N. Padian. 1980. Children's symptom and social functioning self-report scales: comparison of mothers' and children's reports. *Journal of Nervous and Mental Diseases* 168:736–740.

Weitzman, M. 1984. School and peer relations. *Pediatric Clinics of North America* 31:59–70.

Wood, R. E. 1984. Prognosis. In L. M. Taussig, ed., *Cystic fibrosis.* New York: Thieme Stratton.

12. Teenage Pregnancy

Alan Guttmacher Institute. 1981. *Teenage pregnancy: the problem that hasn't gone away.* New York: Institute publication.

Authier, K., and J. Authier. 1982. Interventions with families of pregnant adolescents. In I. R. Stuart and C. F. Wells, eds., *Pregnancy in adolescence—needs, problems, and management.* New York: Van Nostrand Reinhold.

Barrera, M., Jr. 1981. Social support in the adjustment of pregnant adolescents. In B. H. Gottlieb, ed., *Social networks and social support.* Beverly Hills: Sage.

Barret, R. L., and B. E. Robinson. 1982. A descriptive study of teenage expectant fathers. *Family Relations* 31:349–352.

Bierman, B., and R. Streett. 1982. Adolescent girls and mothers: problems in parenting. In I. R. Stuart, and C. F. Wells, eds., *Pregnancy in adolescence—needs, problems, and management.* New York: Van Nostrand Reinhold.

Brooks-Gunn, J., and F. F. Furstenberg. In press. The children of adolescent mothers: physical, academic, and psychological outcomes. *Developmental Review.*

Brown, S. V. 1983. The commitment and concerns of black adolescent parents. *Social Work Research and Abstracts* 19:27–34.

Cartoof, V. G., and L. V. Klerman. In press. Parental consent for abortion: impact of the Massachusetts law. *American Journal of Public Health.*

Colletta, N. 1981. Social support and the risk of maternal rejection by adolescent mothers. *Journal of Psychology* 109:191–197.

Fine, P., and M. Pape. 1982. Pregnant teenagers in need of social networks: diagnostic parameters. In I. R. Stuart and C. F. Wells, eds., *Pregnancy in adolescence—needs, problems, and management.* New York: Van Nostrand Reinhold.

Forrest, J. D., A. I. Hermalin, and S. K. Henshaw. 1981. The impact of family planning clinic programs on adolescent pregnancy. *Family Planning Perspectives* 13:109–116.

Furstenberg, F. F., Jr. 1981. Implicating the family: teenage parenthood and kinship involvement. In T. Oooms, *Teenage pregnancy in a family context—implications for policy.* Philadelphia: Temple University Press.

—— and A. G. Crawford. 1978. Family support: helping teenage mothers to cope. *Family Planning Perspectives* 10:322–333.

Hendricks, L. E., and T. Montgomery. 1983. A Limited population of unmarried adolescent fathers: a preliminary report of their views on fatherhood and the relationship with the mothers of their children. *Adolescence* 18:201–210.

Kellam, S. G. 1978–79. *Consequences of teenage motherhood for mother, child, and family in a black urban community.* Progress reports to National Institute of Child Health and Human Development, July 1978 and June 1979.

Kinard, E. M., and H. Reinherz. 1984. Behavioral and emotional functioning in children of adolescent mothers. *American Journal of Orthopsychiatry* 54:578–594.

Leishman, K. 1980. Teenage mothers are keeping their babies—with the help of their own mothers. *MS* 8:61–67.

Levy, S. B., and W. J. Grinker. 1983. *Choices and life circumstances—an ethnographic study of Project Redirection teens.* New York: Manpower Demonstration Research Corporation.

Lorenzi, M. E., L. V. Klerman, and J. F. Jekel. 1977. School-age parents: how permanent a relationship? *Adolescence* 12:13–22.

Olds, D. L., C. R. Henderson, Jr., M. T. Birmingham, R. Chamberlin, and R. Tatelbaum. 1983. *Final report: prenatal/early infancy project.* National Technical Information Service, U.S. Department of Commerce, Springfield, Virginia.

Perlman, R., and J. Z. Geile. 1983. An unstable triad: dependents' demands, family resources, community supports. In R. Perlman, ed., *Family home care: critical issues for services and policies.* New York: Haworth Press.

Schwab, B. 1983. Some one to always be there. Dissertation, Department of Anthropology, Brandeis University.

Taves, E. 1983. Interview. *Health Education Bulletin* 34:3.

Yale Bush Center in Child Development and Social Policy, Family Support Project. 1983. *Programs to strengthen families: a resource guide.* New Haven.

Zabin, L. S., and S. D. Clark, Jr. 1983. Institutional factors affecting teenagers' choice and reasons for delay in attending a family planning clinic. *Family Planning Perspectives* 15:25–29.

Zelnik, M., and J. F. Kantner. 1980. Sexual activity, contraceptive use and pregnancy among metropolitan-area teenagers, 1971–1979. *Family Planning Perspectives* 12:230–237.

Zitner, R., and S. H. Miller. 1980. *Our youngest parents—a study of the use of support services by adolescent mothers.* New York: Child Welfare League of America.

13. Education of Families for Parenting

Berrueta-Clement, J. R., L. J. Schweinhart, W. S. Barnett, A. S. Epstein, and D. P. Weikart. 1984. *Changed lives: the effects of the Perry Preschool Program on youths through age 19.* Ypsilanti, Michigan: High-Scope Educational Research Foundation.

Caldwell, B. M. 1980. Balancing children's rights and parents' rights. In R.

Haskins and J. J. Gallagher, eds., *Care and education of young children in America: policy, politics, and social science.* Norwood, New Jersey: Ablex.

Children learning about children. Videotape. Program prepared for elementary school health education curriculum. University of Arkansas at Little Rock: Available through author.

Gesell, A., and C. S. Amatruda. 1946. *Developmental diagnosis.* New York: Hoeber.

——and F. Ilg. 1943. *The infant and child in the culture of today.* New York: Harper.

Lazar, I., and R. Darlington. 1982. Lasting effects of early education. *Monographs of the Society for Research in Child Development* 47:1–2.

Ruhrah, J. 1925. *Pediatrics of the past.* New York: Hoeber.

Scales, P. 1981. Sex education in the '70s and '80s: accomplishments, obstacles and emerging issues. *Family Relations* 30:557–566.

White House Conference on the Family. 1982. Final Report. Government Printing Office.

14. The Social-Policy Context for Families Today

Allen, M. 1983. Testimony before Committee on Finance, Senate Hearing on the Administration's Proposals for FY 1984 Spending Reductions, 15 June. Washington, D.C.: Children's Defense Fund.

Berreuta-Clement, J., L. Schweinhart, W. Barnett, and D. Weikart. 1983. *The effects of early educational intervention on crime and delinquency in adolescence and early adulthood.* Ypsilanti: High-Scope Educational Research Foundation.

Blank, H. 1983. *Children and federal child care cuts: a national survey of the impact of federal title XX cuts on state child care systems, 1981–83.* Washington, D.C.: Children's Defense Fund.

Bock, T., and E. Moore. 1981. *Profiles of American youth: demographic influences on ASVAB test performance.* Chicago: National Opinion Research Center.

Brown, L. 1983. Testimony before Subcommittee on Domestic Marketing, Consumer Relations and Nutrition, U.S. House of Representatives, 20 October. Washington, D.C.

Bureau of Labor Statistics. 1983. *Marital and family characteristics of workers.* Washington, D.C.: U.S. Department of Labor.

Center for the Study of Social Policy. 1984a. *The flip-side of black families headed by women: the economic status of black men.* Washington, D.C.: CSSP.

—— 1984b. *Working female-headed families in poverty: three studies of low-income families affected by the AFDC policy changes of 1981.* Washington, D.C.: CSSP.

Children's Defense Fund. 1984. *A children's defense budget: an analysis of the President's FY 1985 budget and children.* Washington, D.C.: CDF.

Coolsen, P. 1982. Unemployment and child abuse. *Caring* 8(4):6–10.

Cummings, J. 1983a. Breakup of black family imperils gains of decades. *New York Times.* 20 November.

—— 1983b. "Heading a family: stories of seven black women. *New York Times* 21 November.

Greenstein, R. 1983. *The effect of the administration's budget, tax and military policies on low-income Americans.* Washington, D.C.: Inter-religious Task Force on U.S. Food Policy.

Havemann, J. 1982. Sharing the wealth: the gap between rich and poor grows wide. *National Journal* 23 October: 1788–95.

Joe, T., and P. Yu. 1984. Black men, welfare and jobs. *New York Times* 22 May.

Kamerman, S. 1984. Child care in the U.S.: since the need is well-documented, what next? Testimony before Select Committee on Children, Youth, and Families, Child Care Hearing, U.S. House of Representatives, Washington, D.C.

Massachusetts Department of Public Health. 1983. *Massachusetts nutrition survey.* Boston.

Metropolitan Insurance Companies. 1984. Alcohol and other drug abuse among adolescents. *Statistical Bulletin* 65(1):4–13.

Miller, C. 1983. *The world economic crisis and the children.* U.S. Case Study prepared for United Nations' Children's Fund. New York.

—— and L. Schorr. 1983. The environmental and policy context for infants and children in the 1980s. Paper at Third Biennial Training Institute, National Center for Clinical Infant Programs. Washington, D.C.

National Center for Health Statistics. 1983a. Advance report of final natility statistics. *Monthly Vital Statistics Reports* 32 (29 December) supplement. Washington, D.C.: DHHS.

—— 1983b. *Health, United States, 1983.* Washington, D.C.: DHHS.

Pierson, D., D. Walker, and T. Tivnan. 1984. A school-based program from infancy to kindergarten for children and their parents. *Personnel and Guidance Journal* 62(8):448–455.

Rescorla, L., S. Provence, and A. Naylor. 1983. Yale Child Welfare Research Program: description and results. In E. Zigler and E. Gordon, eds., *Day care: scientific and social policy issues.* Boston: Auburn House.

Rivlin, A. 1983. Testimony Before Select Committee on Children, Youth, and Families, U.S. House of Representatives, 28 April. Washington, D.C.

Sanders, A. 1984. *The widening gap: the incidence and distribution of infant mortality and low birth weight in the United States, 1978–1982.* Washington, D.C.: Food Research and Action Center.

Schweinhart, L., and D. Weikart. 1980. *Young children grow up: the effects of the Perry Preschool Program on youth through age 15.* Ypsilanti: High-Scope Educational Research Foundation.

Select Panel for the Promotion of Child Health. 1981. *Better health for our children: a national strategy.* 3 vols. Washington, D.C.: SPPCH.

Swartz, K. 1984. Testimony before Subcommittee on Health, U.S. Senate Committee on Finance, 27 April, Washington, D.C.

Trickett, P., N. Apfel, L. Tosenbaum, and E. Zigler. 1982. A five-year follow-up of participants in the Yale Child Welfare Research Program. In E.

Zigler and E. Gordon, eds., *Day care: scientific and social policy issues*. Boston: Auburn House.

U.S. Congress, House Committee on Ways and Means. 1983. *Background material on poverty, 17 October*. Washington, D.C.: committee print.

Acknowledgments

THIS VOLUME grows out of a conference on the family held at Harvard Medical School in the spring of 1984 which brought together experts in child development, pediatrics, education, child psychiatry, business, and social policy. The Robert Wood Johnson Foundation has provided generous support to the editors for teaching and research over the past decade. We gratefully acknowledge the assistance of Reba Gerane West in assembling and preparing the manuscripts for publication. We also thank Edward Gelb for his assistance in planning and assembling the book.

Index